Poultry Production and Management

NIPA® GENX ELECTRONIC RESOURCES & SOLUTIONS P. LTD.
New Delhi-110 034

About the Editors

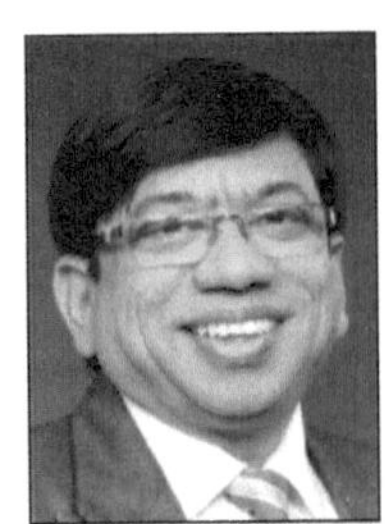

Dr Jeetendra Verma, Born on 19th March 1966, Dr Jeetendra Verma is an eminent business professional in animal health care and nutrition. He graduated from Jabalpur Veterinary College in 1988, MVSc and PhD in Poultry Science from CARI, Izatnagar and a business management graduate from IIM, Kolkata

Dr Verma started his career as Assistant Professor of Poultry Science at Mhow Veterinary College, JNKVV Jabalpur. Later on, he switched from academics to business and joined poultry industry in 1998. Dr Verma has worked with many national and international companies at leadership positions like Nav Maharashtra, Jubilant Organosys, Eli Lilly (Elanco), Delacon Biotechnik etc. Presently he is Market Access Consultant for Asia region for Addicoo, Czech Republic.

He has more than 29 years of experience in the field of Animal Nutrition and Animal Health Care having excellence in managing and leading the companies, exploring and developing new markets, appointing channel partners, accelerating growth & achieving desired marketing and sales goals.

Dr Verma is an honourable member of National Advisory Committee (NAC) constituted by Ministry of Fisheries, Animal Husbandry and Dairying, Govt. of India in 2023 and Research Advisory Committee of ICAR-NIANP, Bangalore.

Dr Verma has received many awards like Frost & Sullivan Award (2005), Aftab Recognition Award (2018), Distinguished Alumni Award 2018 by NDVSU, Jabalpur, Star Anis Award (2016, 2017) by Delacon Biotechnik etc.

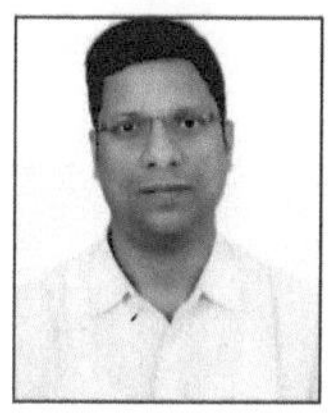

Dr Girraj Goyal, currently holding the post of Incharge, Department of Poultry Science, College of Veterinary Science & Animal Husbandry, NDVSU, Jabalpur. He has obtained his UG degree BVSc. & AH form Mhow Veterinary College, and MVSc & Ph.D degree from Central Avian Research Institute, Izatnagar, Bareilly.

He has more than 13 years of experience in the field of veterinary education, research and extension activities with specialization in Poultry Science. He has established an instructional cum commercial poultry complex at CVSc. & AH, Rewa under ICAR sponsored Experiential Learning Programme. Currently he is associated with ICAR sponsored All India Coordinated Research Project on Poultry Breeding in different capacities including Principal Scientist, Farm Manager etc.

He is working on development of improved varieties of chicken, Japanese quail, Turkey and guinea fowl with special focus on slow growing colour broilers and disease resistance chicken varieties. He is also working on development of development of farmer friendly sustainable technologies for production of enriched meat and eggs with aim to uplift the socio-economic status of the poor and landless farmers, unemployed youth and farm women and to ensure the nutritional security to the deprived classes of the society.

He has published more than 25 research papers in national and international journal. He has authored 5 books & manuals. More than 50 extension & popular articles have been published in his credit in different scientific and social magazines & newspapers. He has been conferred with 5 best paper awards in different international and national conference by reputed scientific societies..

Poultry Production and Management
Recent Trends

Jeetendra Verma
Market Access Consultant (Asia Region)
ADDICOO Group S.R.O., Czech Republic

Girraj Goyal
Assistant Professor & Incharge
Department of Poultry Science
College of Veterinary Science & Animal Husbandry
Nanaji Deshmukh Veterinary Science University
Jabalpur, Madhya Pradesh

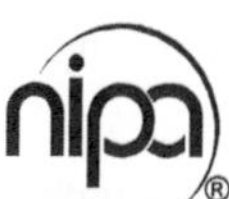

NIPA® GENX ELECTRONIC RESOURCES & SOLUTIONS P. LTD.
New Delhi-110 034

The information provided in this book with articles, images, tables etc has been provided by their respective contributors and neither the editor/s nor the publisher validify the authenticity of the information and the responsibility lies with the respective contributors only.

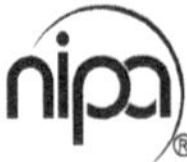

NIPA® GENX ELECTRONIC RESOURCES & SOLUTIONS P. LTD.

101,103, Vikas Surya Plaza, CU Block
L.S.C.Market, Pitam Pura, New Delhi-110 034
Ph : +91 11 27341616, 27341717, 27341718
E-mail: newindiapublishingagency@gmail.com
www: www.nipabooks.com

For customer assistance, please contact
Phone: + 91-11-27 34 17 17
Fax: + 91-11- 27 34 16 16

ISBN: 978-93-58874-09-9

Composed and Designed by NIPA®.

Preface

The book "Poultry Production and Management: Recent Trends," a comprehensive anthology that showcases the latest advancements, emerging paradigms, and indispensable insights in the field of poultry science and management. As the global demand for poultry products continues to rise, it is essential for industry professionals, researchers, and students to understand and adapt to these evolving trends. This book delves into critical aspects of poultry farming, including genetics, nutrition, housing systems, disease management, and sustainability practices, providing a comprehensive overview of the multifaceted landscape of poultry production. In an era marked by rapid technological progress and shifting consumer preferences, this book serves as a guide, helping readers navigate the complex challenges and opportunities that define contemporary poultry farming.

The chapters of this book have been expertly crafted by leading researchers and experts, who have conducted a thorough examination of the most recent findings, innovative applications, and forward-looking ideas in the field of poultry production. The purpose of this book is to equip both beginners and experienced professionals with a comprehensive understanding of the current state of poultry farming, fostering a culture of continuous improvement and innovation. The collaboration of distinguished contributors has been instrumental in the creation of this volume, and their dedication to sharing their knowledge and expertise has not only enriched this compilation but also significantly contributed to the collective wisdom of the poultry industry. We extend our heartfelt gratitude to each contributor for their invaluable contributions.

As editors, our aim is not only to disseminate knowledge but also to inspire curiosity and further exploration in the field of poultry production. We envision this book as a vital resource for academia, industry practitioners, and policymakers, providing a comprehensive guide to navigate the complexities of modern poultry farming. We express our appreciation to the readers for their interest in staying informed about the constantly evolving landscape of poultry production and management. Our hope is that this volume will serve as both a reference guide and a source of inspiration for those committed to advancing the poultry industry.

Editors

Contents

1

Artificial Intelligence (AI) A New Era In Poultry Production

D.N. Desai, M.A. Gole, A.S. Ranade and S.S. Gaikwad

Department of Poultry Science, Mumbai Veterinary College, Parel Maharashtra Animal and Fishery Science University, Nagpur, Maharashtra

At a compound annual growth rate (CAGR) of 7.6%, the global poultry industry expanded from $352.02 billion in 2022 to $378.84 billion in 2023. Global production of chicken meat was projected to reach 103.4 million metric tons in 2023, primarily as a result of rising output in China, India, Brazil, and the US. India is currently the world's second-largest egg producer (138.3 billion eggs in 2022–2023), trailing only China. It is also the world's fifth-largest broiler producer (producing 4.99 metric tons (MT) in 2022–2023), behind China, the United States, Brazil, and the Russian Federation. Two things drove the shift: (1) the government's decision to liberalize the importation of parent chicken stock; and (2) the development of a vertical integration strategy that united major integrators/hatcheries. To sustain and improve such high numbers of production and with the growing concern of the unavailability of cheap and affordable labor, there is an increasing need for humans to rely on technology.

Gadgets and electronic devices are now a necessary part of daily life in the information and technology age. Technology makes it easier for us to go on and complete our daily tasks in an organized way. These days, we carry around a tiny computer called a smartphone that connects us to the internet and other people, providing us with a wealth of possibilities and information. Artificial Intelligence (AI), robotics, sensors, drones, augmented reality, the Internet of Things (IoT), mobile apps, etc. are examples of modern technology that could be used for precision or smart livestock farming. The ability of a computer to carry out tasks that are typically completed by humans and require human intelligence is known as Artificial Intelligence (AI).

Artificial intelligence is the science of making machines that can think like humans. It can do things that are considered "intelligent". Artificial intelligence technology can process large amounts of data in a different way than a human. AI aims to be able to recognize things like patterns, make decisions and make judgments like humans. Artificial intelligence is the simulation of human intelligence processes by machines, especially computer systems.

Several major challenges are present in industrial-scale production, such as high production costs, animal welfare concerns, lack of skilled and trained workers, increased antimicrobial resistance, and environmental adverse effects. However, AI can help to solve the challenges we face today. Poultry industry Most farms collect data manually and then process the data on computers. By 2050, it is predicted that poultry farms will be able to generate 4.1 million data points through various sensors and other devices connected through the Internet of Things. AI-based technology automatically and accurately collects real-time data that can be analyzed in-depth so you can act quickly to optimize your farm's production processes.

AI can learn from data in both supervised and unsupervised ways. In supervised learning, the AI is trained using existing datasets and assigned specific control tasks. For example, predict the expected body weight of a line of broilers under local conditions. Unsupervised learning allows you to categorize the collected data and use cloud resources to detect trends without a specific purpose, analyzing large amounts of data to report results independently. Big data and data mining are the most effective tools for poultry farmers to get the most out of their investment. Few ICT companies focus on forecasting operations based on records and data collected in real time, helping farmers make decisions to optimize farming. Today, high-tech farms involve the use of a wide range of sensors to measure bird body weight, temperature, feed and water intake, humidity, ammonia levels, CO2 levels, and many other parameters. Machines and computer-controlled machines can reduce human interaction with farm birds, reduce sources of disease, and reduce the amount of productive work performed by humans. AI can reduce error rates to low levels and work 24/7 improving agriculture to increase agricultural yields. In the near future, AI may transform the current landscape of traditional industrial agriculture-based Poultry farming into smart poultry or AI-assisted poultry farming.

Applications of Artificial Intelligence in Poultry Industry, Daily Farm Management

Machine learning is poised to revolutionize the future of agricultural management. With the help of machine learning, robots can precisely control various critical parameters required for efficient farm management. AI is more than collecting data. From the data previously stored in the cloud, the information can be processed through data analysis. Using AI to analyze data can make decisions faster, improving farms and efficiency.

For example, robots can be programmed to collect data on management and environmental levels on a farm. This data is processed so that the machine can make a specific decision about the gas. It's a big but repetitive job that affects farm efficiency and productivity. Machine learning and data analytics can handle these tasks efficiently by continuously monitoring farm operations that could otherwise be problematic for humans.

Many universities are evaluating poultry farm management systems using technologies such as Zigbee and Raspberry Pi integrated with wireless sensors and GPRS. These technologies are expected to enter the poultry industry on a larger scale shortly.

Artificial intelligence can also be used in tasks such as feeding, watering and cleaning to streamline and automate these critical tasks. Data analytics is an important function of gathering and analyzing current data to predict future outcomes. For example, tracking and analyzing current data can accurately predict bird weight after 30 days. The implementation of AI in farm management brings efficiency, accuracy, and faster decision-making to the system.

Disease Management

Disease management is extremely important in farming operations because all aspects of farm operations are closely related to it. Implementing machine-based disease management can be difficult because of the diversity of symptoms and the multitude of possible diseases. However, artificial intelligence (AI) is expected to simplify this process in the near future, especially through its role in diagnostics. This is where machine learning and big data come into play, which is the key to effective disease control. With cameras installed on farms, AI can quickly identify problems such as bird predation and cannibalism and quickly notify caretakers so they can make faster decisions and minimize damage. Birds often exhibit unique vocalizations and abnormal behavior during illness. By entering information about such characteristics into the system, the machines can be programmed to immediately alert veterinarians when troubling behavior is detected.

In addition, mobile applications can help pathologists and consultants in confirming the diagnosis. These apps can use mobile cameras to provide better diagnostic insights. However, creating such applications requires a significant amount of expertise. Machine systems within the facility can use this information to diagnose illnesses and quickly notify facility managers when intervention is needed.

In 2012, researchers at the University of Oxford conducted a remarkable experiment called "Chicken Time Warp", "coordinated herd movement can help detect diseases up to a week before they start". Such predictive capabilities can help farmers combat disease-related losses and can be applied to various deadly poultry diseases.

In conclusion, AI-based disease management is promising for the poultry industry as machine learning and big data play a key role in enabling early detection, accurate diagnosis and timely intervention, ultimately leading to better disease management and reduced losses for farmers.

Post-Farm Operations

AI has already made significant advances in poultry production in many developed countries, resulting in significant improvements in efficiency. Companies involved in meat processing are pursuing advanced technologies like artificial intelligence and machine vision to categorize chicken pieces and identify diseased carcasses.The accuracy of AI-controlled machines in detecting muscle mass and bone density makes it possible to automate tasks like bone removal.Layer farming uses artificial intelligence to perform tasks such as egg collection, grading, and the quick identification of good-quality eggs.

By utilizing both machine vision and intelligent automation, the carcass quality and packaging in poultry have undergone significant improvements. Birds can be pre-sorted with precision using spectral imaging systems, as has been demonstrated.

Sensors

In recent years, multimedia technology has made significant advances in terms of content, accuracy and cost-effectiveness. Widely used wireless sensors are found in a variety of fields, including agriculture and environment as well as civil engineering and emergency management (Ruiz-Garcia *et al.*, 2009). While integration in various sectors has been around for a long time, integration in agriculture is a recent development. Initially, the focus was on using these sensors to reduce operational costs and improve animal welfare in the agricultural sector.

Environment Sensors

The environment plays a crucial role in shaping the health, welfare and productivity of broilers, with the humidity level, temperature, and weather being the most significant factors. Moreover, the emission of toxic gases like ammonia and carbon dioxide can have adverse impacts on chicken growth as well as feed conversion and immune responses. Studies have shown that short-term exposure of chickens to high levels of carbon monoxide increases mortality and changes in cardiovascular conditions (Olanrewaju *et al.*, 2008). Therefore, bird welfare is closely linked to the monitoring and regulating of environmental conditions.

Monitoring and control of environmental factors other than temperature are not used in commercial poultry farms, but advances in sensor technology have made it possible to build small environmental regulation systems. For example, these multiple systems can track different parameters such as ambient temperature, air pressure difference, and air velocity in the broiler flock (Bustamante *et al.*, 2017). By evaluating the production systems, their design and performance are automatically evaluated to maintain a good environment for chickens.

In addition, sensors can be integrated to collect data on relative humidity and temperature, as well as ammonia and carbon dioxide (Jackman e*t al.*, 2015). Real-time monitoring of the environment is complemented by sophisticated modeling tools, which can be used to create alert systems that detect any deviations from weight gain. This system can also ensure the health and welfare of the chickens. This approach holds the promise of providing optimal environmental conditions for birds.

Acoustic Sensors

The study of biological sounds generated by living organisms is known as bioacoustical science.Birds social interactions and warning signals are heavily dependent on communication among living organisms. (Corkery *et al.*, 2013). Acoustic studies span from straightforward evaluation of phonological variations to intricate analyses of the characteristics. For example, Zimmerman *et al.* (2000) used basic acoustic parameters such as vocal frequency to identify nutritional deficiencies in broilers and laying hens.

Acoustic analysis has emerged as an important method for evaluating thermal environmental efficiency. Moura *et al.* (2008) conducted a study to evaluate the thermal comfort and performance of broilers by analyzing the amplitude and frequency of sounds. They studied thebird'sbehavioral responses when placed in different environmental conditions. The study found that as the temperature dropped, the amplitude and frequency of the hens' calls increased as they huddled together to protect themselves from the low temperature. However, when the birds were exposed to heat, their calls continued to increase in intensity and frequency. This study shows how acoustic analysis can help understand the health and behavior of broiler chickens under different thermal conditions.

Sound analysis has also been shown to be used during hatching to limit hatch time (the time between the first and last hatched egg). This period has a significant impact on broiler health and performance. Early hatching causes problems such as dehydration and increased mortality, while late hatching reduces hatchability and reduces chick quality. Additionally, differences in hatching time affect chick feeding behavior and increase fear of early hatching males. Therefore, it is important to carefully monitor the late stages of hatching to reduce the risks associated with early hatching and late hatching.

These research studies show the diverse potential of using acoustic analysis to improve house conditions in chickens and to identify behavioral or negative problems. Since sound technology has been around for a long time and it is easy to assess specific parameters, there is a lot of potential for introduction in commercial environments to improve the health and welfare of chickens.

Motion Sensors

Promoting free movement is important to ensure animal welfare. Because it is important that animals have a chance for life. However, many factors related to poultry farming practices, including overcrowding, limited space, and health concerns, restrict bird movement. As a result, the degree of movement or lack of movement accurately reflects the health of the hens. The motion sensor monitored movement patterns in broilers and laying hens. A popular example is the use of piezoelectric crystals to assess gait problems in fattening chickens. It focused on measuring the maximum vertical force exerted on both legs during the weak moments (Naas *et al.*, 2010). With this approach, we were able to identify the asymmetry of peak force between each leg, which explained the irregular gait observed in broiler chickens. These developments represent a significant advance in achieving real-time evaluation of broiler performance (Banerjee*et al.*, 2014).

In summary, motion sensors and related technologies play an important role in assessing and improving chicken welfare. The use of motion sensors offers an opportunity to improve the design and management processes aimed at improving the health of chickens and laying hens, considering motor impairments, and assessing the progress and risk of different construction systems. These data help identify areas for improvement and implement measures that focus on bird welfare and comfort (Daigle *et al.*, 2014).

Sensors for Detection of the Health Status of Birds

Under carefully monitored experimental conditions, wireless devices with body temperature sensors and accelerometers were used to identify bees infected with highly pathogenic avian influenza up to 6 hours before death (Okada *et al.*, 2009). The research team subsequently developed a smart device that uses three-axis wireless accelerometers and radial heat exchangers. To enable early analysis of bird flu symptoms, this improved system transmitted activity and temperature data to wireless sensor nodes. This technology has demonstrated its ability to detect abnormalities caused by the disease twice as fast as using only a body temperature sensor, reaching 100%.

Although these detection devices are difficult to implement in large flocks, they can be used effectively in small populations of resident birds, as a preventive or early detection strategy, especially in high-risk areas. In addition, since temperature fluctuations and decreased activity are common symptoms of various diseases, this simple device can also act as an alarm system to detect other health risks.

Use of Robots in Poultry Farming

Various companies like "Octopus Poultry Robotics" have developed high-tech robots that have made management practices easier for the farmers. These robots (XO, T-MOOV, EASY-LIT) are equipped with advanced communication and navigation systems that facilitate optimal guidance and tracking, just like autonomous vehicles. These robots focus on Reconciling productivity, environment, and animal welfare through continuous litter treatment and environmental and animal monitoring. These robots work completely autonomously thanks to its LIDAR navigation system and on-board cameras.They constantly scarify the litter and spray sanitizers continuously thereby cleaning the litter and reducing ammonia production. They also have various sensors built in their system to monitor the environment for mapping temperature, humidity, and ammonia. Onboard cameras help in the detection, counting, and localization of dead chickens. They are connected to smartphones and tablets providing real-time alerts and data.

As each coin has two sides artificial intelligence also has benefits and drawbacks for the poultry sector.In Nut shell they can summarized are as.

Benefits of Artificial Intelligence

- Use of sensors and vision systems to get real-time data.
- Ability to promptly implement corrective measures and/or alert the farmer.
- Reduce tedious and painstaking manual labor in farms.
- Reduces losses, and improves yield and quality.
- Stores the data for future reference.
- Automatic machine learning.

Drawbacks of Artificial Intelligence

- High initial investment cost.
- Expensive maintenance.
- Requires constant updates.
- Risk of malfunctions.
- It Can't be compared to human judgement.
- Decreased personal touch.
- Increased reliance on technology.
- Loss of traditional skills.

Conclusion

There is strong speculation about the impact of artificial intelligence on the poultry industry. In the near future, we expect AI to revolutionize the poultry sector and have a positive impact by improving efficiency and accuracy at all levels of the industry. Many companies have begun to explore the application of AI throughout their value chain and actively implement AI solutions.

Artificial intelligence has great potential in the poultry industry as it faces many challenges that would be impossible without the introduction of machinery and equipment. Adopting new technologies will help to optimize production systems and efficiency, making poultry and eggs more valuable to consumers. In general, the progress of AI in the poultry industry will encourage positive changes and open up new opportunities for the sector.

References

20th Livestock Census. All India Report. Ministry of Fisheries, Animal Husbandry & Dairying. Department of Animal Husbandry & Dairying. Animal HusbandryStatistics Division, Krishi Bhawan, New Delhi, 2019.

Banerjee D, Daigle CL, Dong B, Wurtz K, Newberry RC, Siegford JM, et al. Detection of jumping and landing force in laying hens using wireless wearable sensors. Poultry Science. 2014;93(11):2724-2733.

Bustamante E, Calvet S, Estelles F, Torres AG, Hospitaler A. Measurement and numerical simulation of single-sided mechanical ventilation in broiler houses. Biosystems Engineering. 2017; 160:55-68.

Corkery G, Ward S, Kenny C, Hemmingway P. Incorporating smart sensing technologies into the poultry industry. Journal of World's Poultry Research. 2013;3(4):106-128.

Daigle CL, Banerjee D, Montgomery RA, Biswas S, Siegford JM. Moving GIS research indoors: Spatiotemporal analysis of agricultural animals. PLoS One. 2014;9(8):102-107.

Dwivedi YK, Hughes L, Ismagilova E, Aarts G, Coombs C, Crick T, et al. Artificial Intelligence (AI): Multidisciplinary perspectives on emerging challenges, opportunities, and agenda for research, practice and policy. International Journal of Information Management. 2021; 57:101994.

https://www.octopusbiosafety.com/en/home

Ilager S, Muralidhar R, Buyya R. Artificial intelligence (ai)-centric management of resources in modern distributed computing systems. In 2020 IEEE Cloud Summit, 2020, 1-10.

Jackman P, Ward S, Brennan L, Corkery G, McCarthy U. Application of wireless technologies to forward predict crop yields in the poultry production chain. Agricultural Engineering International: CIGR Journal. 2015;17(2):25- 29.

Løtvedt P, Jensen P. Effects of hatching time on behavior and weight development of chickens. PloS One. 2014;9(7):186-188.

Moura DJ, Naas ID, Alves EC, Carvalho TM, Vale MM, Lima KA. Noise analysis to evaluate chick thermal comfort. Scientia Agricola. 2008; 65:438-43.

Naas ID, Paz IC, Baracho MD, Menezes AG, Lima KA, Bueno LG, et al. Assessing locomotion deficiency in broiler chicken. Scientia Agricola. 2010; 67:129-135.

Nielsen BL, Juul-Madsen HR, Steenfeldt S, Kjaer JB. Feeding activity in groups of newly hatched broiler chicks: effects of strain and hatching time. Poultry Science. 2010;89(7):1336-44.

Okada H, Itoh T, Suzuki K, Tsukamoto K. Wireless sensor system for detection of avian influenza outbreak farms at an early stage. In SENSORS, 2009 the Institute of Electrical and Electronics Engineers. 2009; 10:1374- 1377.

Okada H, Suzuki K, Kenji T, Itoh T. Applicability of wireless activity sensor network to avian influenza monitoring system in poultry farms. Journal of Sensor Technology. 2014; 4:18-23.

Olanrewaju HA, Thaxton JP, Dozier Iii WA, Purswell J, Collier SD, Branton SL. Interactive effects of ammonia and light intensity on hematochemical variables in broiler chickens. Poultry Science. 2008;87(7):1407-1414.

Rowe E, Dawkins MS, Gebhardt-Henrich SG. A systematic review of precision livestock farming in the poultry sector: Is technology focussed on improving bird welfare?. Animals. 2019;9(9):614-615.

Ruiz-Garcia L, Lunadei L, Barreiro P, Robla JI. A review of wireless sensor technologies and applications in agriculture and food industry: state of the art and current trends. Sensors. 2009;9(6):4728-4750.

Tefera M. Acoustic signals in domestic chicken (*Gallus gallus*): a tool for teaching veterinary ethology and implication for language learning. Ethiopian Veterinary Journal. 2012;16(2):77-84.

Thornton G. 16 innovations to change poultry production. Poultry Tech Summit, Atlanta, 5-7, November 2018, WATT Global Media event, 2018, p. 63.

Zimmerman PH, Koene P, van Hooff JA. The vocal expression of feeding motivation and frustration in the domestic laying hen, *Gallus gallusdomesticus*. Applied Animal Behaviour Science. 2000;69(4):265-273.

2

Cage-Free Farming A Pathway to Sustainable Egg Production & Enhanced Animal Welfare

Rokade J.J., Prasad Wadajkar, Nagabhushan K. Nagesh Sonale, Monika M. and Tiwari A.K.

ICAR-Central Avian Research Institute, Bareilly, Uttar Pradesh-243122

In recent years, the global agricultural landscape has witnessed a paradigm shift towards more sustainable and ethical practices, with a particular focus on the well- being of animals. One such notable transformation is evident in the egg production industry, where traditional methods are being reconsidered in favour of more humane alternatives. Cage-free farming has emerged as a promising path, not only for meeting the demands of a conscientious consumer base but also for addressing concerns related to animal welfare. Cage-free farming represents a departure from conventional egg production systems that confine laying hens to small, restrictive cages. Instead, it offers an environment that allows hens to express natural behaviors, such as walking, spreading their wings, and nesting. This shift signifies a broader commitment to ensuring the physical and psychological health of animals involved in the food production chain. As the industry navigates these changes, it becomes imperative to explore the implications of cage-free farming on both egg production and animal welfare.

Animal Welfare Concepts

There is a widely shared agreement on the idea of animal welfare, indicating a balanced state of well-being for the animal in relation to its environment. In practice, this can be understood as providing them sufficient health and comfort, as well as avoiding stress of any order. Ultimately, inadequate housing for broilers results in a direct decline in production. This prompts the consideration that health, welfare, and productivity are intricately intertwined. A comprehensive examination of animal welfare was previously assembled by fox (1994), focusing on factors such as welfare determinants, cognitive ethology, self-awareness, and the consciousness, emotions, and suffering of animals. Duncan & petherick (1991) differentiated needs from desires, sensing from detecting, and perception from learning and awareness, among other concepts. More recently, some authors support the idea that welfare is mainly (dawkins, 1990) or solely (duncan, 1993) dependent on what the animal feels more than its response. Currently, intensive poultry production places significant emphasis on meeting the requirements for animal welfare. Issues like beak trimming, stocking density, free access to feed, heat stress, and air pollutants have gained significance, leading to regulatory measures in various countries. Simultaneously, the absence of effective evaluations of animal welfare poses a significant challenge for developing welfare regulations and advancing our understanding of animal well-being. It's important to note that welfare extends beyond the mere avoidance of cruelty or 'unnecessary suffering,' challenging common assumptions. However, the understanding of animal welfare goes beyond a simple assessment and can be elucidated through different states.

Physical state is traditionally emphasized, focused primarily on the physiological well-being of animals. Mcglone (1993) asserted that an animal experiences poor welfare only when physiological systems are disrupted to the extent that survival or reproduction is compromised. Mcglone holds an extreme perspective, asserting that welfare is subpar only when a physical problem hampers survival or reproduction. Fraser and broom (1990) offer a broader definition, stating that welfare characterizes the state of an animal concerning its efforts to adapt to its environment.

Mental state is also recognized as pivotal in animal welfare. Duncan (1993) contends that neither health, lack of stress, nor fitness alone is sufficient to determine good welfare; rather, welfare hinges on what animals feel.

Naturalness another dimension is naturalness, which pertains to an animal's ability to fulfill its innate needs and desires. Frustration resulting from the non-fulfillment of these needs adversely affects welfare. This aspect implies that optimal welfare is contingent on animals leading a 'natural' life and expressing their evolved behavioral patterns. Some behaviours have evolved as an adaptation to deal with an adverse situation (distress calls in isolation, fleeing from a predator and so on).

Progression Towards Cage free-was Motivated by the Following Factors

Growing concern for animal welfare, spanning domestic pets, farm animals, and wildlife, has given rise to the concept of "Animal rights." This heightened awareness extends across various animal categories, indicating a societal shift towards ethical treatment. In the post-war era, the primary focus was on fulfilling the population's basic needs, as seen in measures like egg rationing in the UK until 1954. As living standards improved, consumers began prioritizing quality, with humane production practices becoming a symbol of product excellence. Public concern evolution created a market opportunity, prompting poultry equipment companies to develop technologies facilitating mass production of cage eggs. Consequently, costs associated with producing cage-free eggs decreased, approaching those of cage eggs. However, consideration for animal welfare varies along a spectrum. While many consumers value humane practices, a substantial price difference between cage-free and conventional eggs may hinder widespread adoption. If the cost of cage-free eggs were comparable to cage eggs, the majority of consumers would likely choose cage-free options. The graph illustrating the global development of cage-free farming mirrors changing consumer preferences and industry practices.

Evolution of Housing Systems

Chickens, historically housed in floor systems for over 8,000 years since domestication, have experienced shifts towards more humane housing systems due to evolving awareness. Backyard chickens, still common globally, are typically floor-housed with varying space provisions. The standard housing system for egg production shifted to conventional cages in the 1930s, a pivotal moment in the industrialization of the egg production sector. These cages brought essential benefits to egg producers, including more efficient space utilization, fully automated processes, easier management, superior hygiene, lower infectious disease incidence, reduced feed consumption, and lower production costs. While cage systems proved successful, they faced early criticism. By the 1960s, the significance of animal welfare was growing in europe, and cages came under scrutiny for constraining bird movement and impeding the natural expression of behavioral patterns in laying hens. Furnished cages – also known as enriched, colony or modified cages – were first developed in the 1980s. Furnished cages were designed as an effort to integrate the merits of both conventional cages, focusing on hygiene and production efficiency, and cage-free systems. In addition to offering more space per hen compared to traditional cages, furnished cages typically include amenities such as perches, nests, scratching areas, and nail shorteners, incorporating some features associated with cage-free environments. The provision of specific elements in furnished cages may vary from country to country or region to region. While furnished cages are acknowledged to enhance hens' behavioral expression compared to conventional cages and improve their physical well-being, concerns have been raised about the limitations in expressing certain natural behaviors due to inherent constraints in caged environments, such as limited locomotion, ground-scratching, wing-flapping, and flying.

Ongoing Pressure on Furnished Cages

Despite EU-wide legislation permitting furnished cages, several member states have prohibited all types of cages for egg production, with others planning similar bans. Industry stakeholders are steering egg production towards a 'post-cage era,' not only in the EU but also in the USA and various other countries. According to Compassion in World Farming's 2020 Egg Track Report, numerous major egg producers, retailers, food service companies, and hotel chains, including global corporations, have committed to eliminating cage eggs from their supply chains. This shift has led to a significant reduction in the share of eggs produced in cages in recent years, with the EU dropping from 68% in 2008 to 48% in 2020, and cage-free flocks in the USA increasing from 5% in 2009 to an estimated 29% in 2026.

Economic Impact of Welfare Requirements

The economic impact of welfare requirements, influenced by Council Directive 1999/74/EC, has reshaped egg production in the EU. This directive mandated changes in cage space per hen, leading to increased production costs in 2003 and the eventual ban on conventional cages in 2012. The cost of egg production in non-cage systems (barn/aviary, free-range, or organic) or furnished cages has risen significantly, with a 23% increase in the EU post-2012 compared to pre-2012 cage production. Similar cost differentials are observed in the USA, where producing eggs in furnished cages is 13% higher than in conventional cages and aviary production is 36% more expensive.

Cage Free System

- Cage-free egg production, characterized by hens not confined to cages, encompasses various systems offering more space for movement.
- Stocking density ranges from 10 to 15 birds/m^2 for pullets and 9 to 13 birds/m^2 for adult birds.
- The minimum indoor space is 1,100 cm^2,
- Flock sizes can vary from small-scale to large-scale production, involving hundreds to tens of thousands of birds.

Advantages of Cage-Free Farming

1. **Improved animal welfare:** Cage-free systems provide animals with more space to move and engage in natural behaviors, promoting better overall welfare compared to traditional cage systems. Hens, for example, can express more natural behaviors such as nesting and dust bathing.
2. **Consumer perception and market demand:** Many consumers are increasingly concerned about the ethical treatment of animals and are willing to pay a premium for products from cage-free systems. Meeting this demand can enhance a farm's market competitiveness and profitability.
3. **Reduced risk of disease spread:** Cage-free systems may reduce the risk of disease transmission compared to crowded cage environments. Improved ventilation and space can contribute to healthier animals, potentially lowering the need for antibiotics and mitigating disease outbreaks.
4. **Environmental benefits:** Cage-free systems may have positive environmental impacts, as they can allow for more sustainable waste management practices. The distribution of manure over a larger area can aid in nutrient recycling and reduce the environmental impact of concentrated waste.
5. **Compliance with animal welfare standards:** Many countries and regions are adopting or considering regulations that mandate improved living conditions for farm animals. Transitioning to cage-free systems helps farms comply with evolving animal welfare standards and regulations.

Challenges of Cage-Free Farming

1. **Higher Initial Investment and Operating Costs:** Transitioning to cage-free systems often require significant upfront investment in infrastructure and may involve higher ongoing operating costs. This can pose a financial challenge for some farmers.
2. **Space and Resource Constraints:** Cage-free systems require more space, which may be a limiting factor for farms with limited land availability. Additionally, providing adequate resources such as feed, water, and nesting areas for animals in larger spaces can be challenging.
3. **Egg Quality and Safety Concerns:** Cage-free systems may present challenges in maintaining egg quality and safety. For example, the increased contact between hens and their environment can lead to higher risks of contamination, requiring more stringent measures for hygiene and disease prevention.

4. **Transition Period Challenges:** The transition from conventional cage systems to cage-free farming can be stressful for both farmers and animals. Managing this transition, including retraining staff and acclimating animals to the new system, poses practical challenges.
5. **Potential for Aggressive Behavior Among birds:** In cage-free systems, there is a risk of increased aggression and pecking among animals due to the larger social groups. Farmers need to implement effective strategies to manage social dynamics and prevent injurious behaviors among the animals.

Housing Systems of Cage Free Farming

1. **Single-**Tier/Flat Deck/ Floor Housing System Flat-deck systems typically have only one tier and are the simplest form of barn housing for laying hens. Flock sizes in single-tier systems can range from hundreds to tens of thousands of hens the characteristic features of this system include At least one third of the floor must be solid and covered with litter (LayWel, 2006) there is a central raised area (the tier) with a slatted floor on which feeders, nests and perches are placed (Nicol *et al.*, 2017). A manure pit or a manure removal system is normally placed underneath the central raised slatted area. The nest boxes are usually placed over the slatted floor. Nest boxes are usually covered with an artificial grass bottom or litter and eggs can be collected automatically or manually. Nests can be individual or for groups of hens. Perches are usually placed in A-frames on the slatted floor (LayWel, 2006) or suspended from the ceiling.
2. **Multi-**Tier/Aviary Aviaries, also referred to as multi-tier systems, are structural accommodations that enable hens to move freely across several tiers, with EU legislation allowing a maximum of four tiers (Windhorst, 2017). Aviaries exhibit diverse designs, emphasizing the efficient use of vertical space within the barn. Perches, feeders, drinkers, and nest boxes are strategically distributed across multiple tiers, their specific placement dictated by the aviary design. Similar to other barn systems, the maximum allowable stocking density in aviaries is 9 birds/ m^2 of usable area. While flock size may vary from small to large-scale production, aviaries are commonly utilized in large-scale barn egg production due to their significant setup costs.

   Well-designed aviary systems aim to support essential behaviors for hens, including:

- Perching and roosting on aerial perches;
- Performing nest seeking and egg-laying behaviours in collective nests;
- Using feed and water lines;
- Pecking, scratching and dust-bathing when on the ground littered area

Flat deck systems and aviaries can be equipped with covered verandas (also sometimes called "winter gardens"). These are covered areas adjacent to the main barn, which offer natural light and are accessed via pop-holes. Verandas provide birds with additional space to dust-bathe in litter, forage if enrichments are provided, and enjoy natural light and, often, fresh air (CIWF, 2012a).

3. **Mobile Sheds-** Mobile sheds are a housing system most frequently used for smaller free-range flocks (typically 200 – 2,000 hens) and in organic egg production. They function like fully equipped "polytunnels" on skids or wheels and use natural ventilation, with an internal layout similar to flat-deck (single tier) housing systems (Nicol *et al.*, 2017). The distinctive feature of these systems is the suspended slatted flooring. Mobile poultry houses are methodically relocated and rotated among different fields or pastures.

Best Practices to Optimize Hens Welfare

1. Feed & Water Welfare

Impacts of feed and water comprise the three main elements namely suitability, quantity and accessibility. Among the three factors, the design of the housing system can impact accessibility, while management decisions play a crucial role in determining suitability and quantity. It is essential for laying hens to have unrestricted access to sufficient feed and water. Access to feed and water can be facilitated by splitting hens into groups. The composition of feed plays a significant role in influencing health parameters, with a notable impact on issues such as injurious feather pecking. Insufficient fiber or amino acid content in the diet has been associated with a higher likelihood of severe feather pecking, prompting the potential need for fiber supplementation, as suggested by Nicol *et al.* (2017). Providing hens with the opportunity to forage by scattering grains and fibrous feed on the ground allows them to complement their diets and engage in natural behaviors. Adding insoluble grit to the diet can also contribute to a healthy digestive system.

2. Physical Characteristics & Environment

The following environmental parameters have a direct impact on animal health and welfare, as well as on productivity:

a. **Lighting regime,** The Laying Hen Directive states that the lighting pattern for laying hens must "include an adequate uninterrupted period of darkness lasting, by way of indication, about one third of the day, so that the hens may rest". The requirement for a sufficient period of uninterrupted darkness stems from the understanding that daylight encourages certain active behaviors, and hens need a dedicated time for resting. Systems incorporating outdoor access or covered verandas can facilitate exposure to natural daylight.

b. **Temperature:** Regarding temperature and humidity, hens are most comfortable within the range of 18 to 27 degrees Celsius (Wageningen UR, 2004). A thermo-neutral zone, where they are very comfortable, is identified between 20-25 degrees Celsius (Nicol *et al.*, 2017). Adequate ventilation, whether natural or forced, is crucial to ensure the removal of excessive heat, odors, and humidity from the hen house. This helps maintain optimal conditions for the well-being of the hens. Heating Should Be Used In Colder Climates, As Below 10 Degrees Celsius Hens Start Suffering From Cold Stress (Ibid.)

c. **Air Quality:** The Presence Of Dust, Endotoxins From Bacteria, Ammonia, Etc. Influences Not Only Animal Health, But Also The Environmental Impact Of The Farm And The Health Of Operators (See Section 6). Aviary systems employing belt removal of manure frequently achieve superior air quality compared to systems utilizing manure pits, as commonly seen in most single-deck housing. However, Depending On Outside Temperature, Maintaining Good Air Quality Parameters Can Be Problematic Irrespective Of Housing System (Nicol *et al.*, 2017).

3. Freedom Choose Among Different Functional Areas

Different Functional Areas Include Outdoor Access, Perching Area, Dustbathing Area And Nesting Areas May Be Provided Within The Covered Areas Or House The Possibility To Choose Between Different Environments Can Promote Natural Behaviours, Which Can In Turn Reduce The Risk Of Developing Abnormal Behaviours. Outdoor Access To Birds Provide Opportunities For Foraging And Thus Reduce The Incidence Of Feather Pecking (Lambton *et al.*, 2010) Foraging Is A Way For Hens To Complement Their Diet With Sources Of Food Found On The Range (Insects, etc Access

To Outdoors In Early Ages Exposes To Endemic Disease Is Beneficial In Long Term In Getting Immunity in later stages of hens life (CIWF, 2010). The outdoor access may be through the pope holes. Nest boxes : well secluded nest boxes can reduce pre laying stress and promote nest building capacity (Struelens *et al.*, 2008). Provision of nest boxes at accurate position and 1 box for 5 birds reduce chance of floor eggs (Nicol *et al.*, 2017).

4. Enrichments

Litter quality: is essential to keep hens in good health an encouraging foraging and dustbathing, the litter should be dry and friable throughout the laying cycle has been defined as "the single most important enrichment to reduce the risk of feather pecking (FeatherWel, undated). **Enrichments** can be introduced to further encourage natural behaviours, particularly in the indoor environment. Enrichments in such systems encompass items like straw bales, pecking blocks, appropriate hanging items (such as edible or destructible objects), as well as grain and grubs. Elevated welfare standards usually mandate the inclusion of at least two types of suitable environmental enrichment within the housing. Enrichments need to be provided in sufficient quantity for all birds to be able to access them.

5. Health

Immune functions: Hens kept in non-cage systems have a strong immune function. In particular, systems that offer access to the outdoors from a young age can boost immunity through exposure to endemic diseases (Nicol *et al.*, 2017). Immune function can also be boosted by feed supplementation with some types of probiotics that promote gut health (ibid.).

Skeletal health: The layout and design of perches plays a role in the incidence of keel bone fractures. Laying hens are motivated to perch, especially during darkness periods (Nicol *et al.*, 2017), freedom of movement and access to perches can improve bone strength (Nicol *et al.*, 2017), the greater movement of birds may result in more fractures due to collisions with hard objects. The keel bone is particularly susceptible to damage/deformation, with the pressure applied to it during perching and landings a notable risk soft-perches i.e. metal or wooden perches covered with approximately 3 mm thickness of soft polyurethane and/ or ramps or 'stepped' slats are preferable

Foot disorders: foot disorders is due contact with wet litters and inappropriate perches, wet litter can lead to hyperkeratosis and eventually bumblefoot, so litter should be dry, clean and friable. inappropriate perches leads footpad dermatitis (bumblefoot) To reduce the risk of injury and infection, the EFSA

(2015) recommends the use of perches made (or wrapped with) soft materials to improve grip; additionally, perches with a square section and 3-6cm

Infectious and parasitic diseases: With all its advantages, cage-free housing results in exposure to a wide range of pathogens, Avian influenza is of concern in this context during periods of outbreaks among wild birds. The mitigating strategies include Reducing contact with wild birds (especially waterfowl), foxes, and other potential vectors (CIWF, 2016a). Feed should not be stored or made available in range areas. In all systems, suitable biosecurity measures must be in place to prevent infectious disease outbreaks, and good hygiene measures can help to prevent disease from entering a holding. Parasites internal (coccidia, worms), external (red mites, lices) infestation can cause severs bird health and welfare issues. Red mite infestations can lead to injurious feather pecking. Hen houses can be regularly treated against red mites and both hens and eggs should be regularly checked for signs of infestation.

Hygiene: In terms of general hygiene, the regular cleaning and disinfecting of fittings such as nest boxes, maintenance of litter and range areas, and regulation of temperature and ventilation, are important to help safeguard the hens' health and welfare.

6. Stockmanship & Handling

Stockpersons should be trained to correctly and calmly handle the animals and to recognise signs of decreased welfare. This requires an understanding of normal and abnormal behaviour. While the housing system may facilitate the ease of inspection, routine management practices are fundamentally independent of the housing system

7. Stocking Rate

Stocking rate is defined as the number of birds allowed or present per unit area (Nicol *et al.*, 2017). laying hens have the tendency to carry out specific behaviours, such as feeding, or dustbathing all together at the same time (Collins *et al.*, 2010). An increased risk of damp litter and plumage damage at higher stocking densities, and higher levels of corticosterone, a stress hormone (Kang *et al.*, 2016; Steenfeldt and Nielsen, 2015) Ideal stocking density should be 6.17 birds/m2 (European legislation), 7.15 birds per m2 (Global Animal Partnership, 2017), 6.2 birds per m2 (AGW Animal Welfare Approved), The German label "Für mehr Tierschutz" (standard and premium) allows a maximum stocking density of 7 birds/m2. LEI Wageningen calculated that husbandry systems should not exceed 4.5/m2 if birds are to be provided the opportunity to perform their full behavioural repertoire (Wageningen UR project team Houden van Hennen, 2004).

Key Behaviours in Cage Free Farming

1. Nesting Behaviour

Hens are highly motivated to find a nest when they are about to lay an egg. Hens deprived of nests show signs of frustration for one to 1½ hours before the egg is due to be laid. These signs include stereotypic pacing, increased aggression, displacement preening, restlessness, vacuum nesting and a specific vocalization called the gackel-call when hen retains egg for additional period in seeking nest may develop additional layer of calcium. There is a widespread acceptance that preventing hens from performing pre-laying behaviour is a severe welfare concern and that providing hens with a suitable nest site is an essential welfare requirement (Jendral, 2008). In cage-free systems, hens typically have multiple nest boxes to choose from and studies show they will inspect many potential nest sites before making a choice (Meijsser & Hughes, 1989. In free-run egg farms provide 20 nests for every 100 hens (BC SPCA), The cage-free guidelines adopted by UEP (2010), recommend 9 ft2 (.84 m2) of community nest space per 100 hens.

2. Perching Behaviour

Modern egg laying hens retain the strong perching instinct that is seen in their ancestor, the red jungle fowl. Perching helps to conserve body heat and maintain bone volume and strength Hens use perches of different heights for different activities – they will stand and walk on lower perches but prefer to perch higher off the ground, especially when sleeping. Research demonstrates that when hens are provided the option of different perch heights, they will choose the highest perches available at night Higher perches also allow vulnerable hens to escape the more assertive ones, reducing the potential of injury from feather pecking

3. Dustbathing

Dustbathing is a natural behaviour which helps to remove stale oil and damaged feathers to keep hens' plumage in good condition (Olsson & Keeling, 2005) Research indicates that dustbathing leads to pleasure and is therefore important for animal welfare. Animal welfare and behavior experts agree that welfare should be more than just the avoidance of suffering (Widowski & Duncan, 2000). Indeed, expressing behaviours that encourage a positive affective state is part of good welfare and overall well-being.

4. Foraging

Despite easy access to a constant supply of feed, caged hens still retain the natural motivation to forage. Studies show that they will choose to forage rather than just eat the feed available in a feeder (Dawkins, 2015).feather pecking is a type of misdirected foraging behavior (Dixon *et al.*, 2010), providing a foraging substrate is important for reducing the risk of injurious pecking. The wire flooring in battery and furnished cages hinders hens from engaging in foraging and scratching behaviors. The resulting lack of exercise can lead to weak bones, and the lack of opportunity to scratch in the ground can cause overgrown claws (Lay *et al.*, 2011), which can break off easily, causing open, bleeding wounds and increased susceptibility to infection. Research shows that cage-free hens display more foraging behavior and walk more than hens confined to furnished cages (Rodenberg *et al.*, 2008).

In fact, they will spend 50 to 70 percent of their time foraging when given outdoor access.

5. Exploratory Behavior

Like other animals, hens are naturally inquisitive and strongly motivated to explore their environment to gather information and this behavior is important for their overall well-being and health. Animals do not just react to stimuli, they are 'agents' who initiate interactions with their environment. Exploration is an expression of this agency and when it is suppressed it can reduce the range of behaviors performed, negatively affect an animal's emotional state and increase fear and anxiety (Špinka & Wemelsfelder, 2011). Cage-free housing systems, particularly those with outdoor access, can offer far more complexity and choices to stimulate a wider range of behavioral activity and movements including exploration (Rodenberg *et al.*, 2005)

Welfare Disadvantages of Cage-Free and Solutions

1. Injurious Pecking

Feather pecking and cannibalism, together called injurious pecking. these are foraging pecks that have been redirected toward feathers, overcrowding, barren environments, lack of loose litter, lack of foraging opportunity (Dixon, 2008), lack of perches during early rearing, and the genetic strain of the hen Feather pecking has also been associated with fearfulness, and studies have found caged hens to be more fearful than hens in cage-free systems. (Rodenberg *et al.*, 2005)

Solutions

Genetic: Select more docile breeds and strains that have a lower propensity to develop feather pecking

Early-life experiences: Introduce birds to pecking and foraging material at an early age early access to loose litter scattering grain or feed into loose litter for young chicks can help reduce injurious pecking (Knierim *et al.*, 2008) Avoid unnecessary changes to the hen's diet and environment

Environment and management: Provide hens with access to pasture or another complex environment. Provide a proper, nutritious diet, accessible feeders and drinkers, perches and adequate lighting and heating Reduce stocking density or organize hens in more natural social groups.

2. Disease

Exposure Cage-free birds-closer contact with feaces-exposed to pathogens Hens raised on litter may have higher mortality due to viral diseases, such as Marek's disease and Newcastle disease, and to coccidiosis, a parasitic disease which attacks the hen's gut (Lay *et al.*, 2011) Eggs laid on litter- direct contact with feaces-contamination of eggs.

Solutions: Regular monitoring, encourage hens to lay eggs in nest boxes and defecate over slats, Better managemental practices

3. Injuries

Cage-free hens are more prone to keel bone fractures and deformation, and are at higher risk of injury when jumping from perch to perch.

Solutions: Ensure the hen housing system is designed to reduce the incidence of bone deformation, fractures and foot infections. Provide hens with access to perches at a young age. Select breeds that have stronger bones and are more resistant to injury.

4. Air Quality Litter-based systems emit higher levels of ammonia and dust than cage systems (Rodenberg *et al.*, 2005).

Factors Influencing Ammonia Accumulation

Amount of manure stored in a housing system Temperature, moisture, litter, ventilation rate, air velocity, animal weight and animal density also affect the level of this harmful gas (Nimmermark, Lund, Gustafsson & Eduard, 2009) Increased ammonia -inflammation of eye, respiratory problems, decreases feed intake, reduced body weight (Nimmermark *et al.*, 2009).

Solutions: Position feeders and drinkers over slatted areas and limit access to the litter area during the night (Groot Koerkamp *et al.*, 1998) Encourage hens to dustbathe and forage in litter during the day through the provision of suitable substrates Install or improve the barn ventilation system.

Scope For Cage Free Eggs

The cage-free egg movement is gaining momentum globally, driven by concerns about animal welfare, sustainability, and food safety. While conventional battery cages remain the dominant egg production system in many countries, cage-free alternatives are rapidly growing in popularity. This trend is particularly relevant in India, the world's second-largest egg producer, and other developing nations where egg consumption is on the rise.

Indian Scenario

Current status: India's egg industry is dominated by battery cages, accounting for over 95% of production. However, consumer awareness about animal welfare issues is growing, and several major food retailers and restaurant chains have committed to sourcing cage-free eggs.

Drivers of Growth: Rising disposable incomes, increasing urbanization, and westernization of dietary habits are driving egg consumption in India. Additionally, initiatives by animal welfare organizations and government support for alternative farming systems are creating a favorable environment for cage- free production.

Challenges: High infrastructure costs, limited consumer awareness, and the lack of a robust certification system pose challenges for the growth of the cage-free segment.

Global Scenario

Increased Demand: The expected expansion of the worldwide cage-free egg market is forecasted to reach $26.7 billion by 2025, reflecting a compound annual growth rate (CAGR) of 12.3%. This growth is driven by factors such as rising consumer awareness, animal welfare regulations, and ethical sourcing commitments by major food companies.

Regional Variations: Europe and North America are at the forefront of the cage- free movement, with bans or phase-outs on battery cages already in place in several countries. However, the Asian and Latin American markets are still dominated by conventional cages, offering significant growth potential for cage- free alternatives

Sustainability Concerns: Cage-free systems generally have a lower environmental impact than battery cages due to reduced manure production and antibiotic use. Additionally, they can improve worker safety and animal welfare.

Conclusion

The transition to cage-free farming represents a significant stride towards creating a more ethical and sustainable future for egg production. Through an exploration of this agricultural paradigm shift, it becomes evident that cage-free systems offer a compelling pathway to address concerns related to both animal welfare and consumer expectations. The documented benefits of cage-free farming include providing laying hens with the opportunity to engage in natural behaviors, contributing to their physical and psychological well-being. In response to consumers placing a growing emphasis on ethical considerations in their buying choices, the egg production industry must adjust to meet these changing expectations. While acknowledging the positive aspects of cage-free farming, it is essential to recognize the challenges associated with this transition. These challenges range from initial investment costs to the need for robust management practices to ensure the optimal performance of laying hens in cage-free environments. However, as technology, research, and industry expertise continue to advance, these challenges are likely to be addressed, paving the way for a more widespread adoption of cage- free systems. As we move forward, it is imperative for stakeholders in the egg production sector, including farmers, policymakers, and consumers, to collaborate in fostering an environment where ethical and sustainable practices are not only encouraged but also economically viable. The evidence presented in this document suggests that cage-free farming holds promise not only in meeting the growing demand for ethically produced eggs but also in shaping a more compassionate and resilient food production system. In conclusion, the exploration of cage-free farming underscores the interconnectedness of animal welfare, industry sustainability, and consumer preferences.

3

Antibiotic Residue in Poultry Meat

Kshemankar Shrman and Gyansagar Kushwaha

Department of Pharmacology and Toxicology
College of Veterinary Science and Animal Husbandry, Nanaji Deshmukh Veterinary and Animal Sciences University, Jabalpur, Madhya Pradesh

Poultry has grown significantly over the last few decades; nevertheless, as production has increased, the usage of specific medications and feed additives has become essential for illness prevention, treatment, and growth promotion. Around the world, broiler chickens are regarded as one of the main sources of meat. Poultry consumption has increased by more than 100% in the last few decades, from 13% of total meat consumption in 1965 to 28% in 2015. All around the world, but especially in emerging and Asian nations, there is a growing need for chicken meat. The amount of poultry meat consumed worldwide increased from 11 kg per person in 2000 to 14.4 kg in 2011, with predictions that it will reach 17.2 kg per person by 2030. An estimated 108.5 million tonnes of poultry meat were produced in 2014, of which 95.5 to 96 million tonnes came from chickens. The farmer is under constant pressure to produce poultry in the shortest amount of time with the highest yield due to an increase in demand. With the use of contemporary technologies, production may now be completed in six to seven weeks. Better farm health management techniques, feed formulation, and genetic selection are all responsible for this progress along with the use of disease-preventive medicines.

The use of antibiotics, such as tetracycline and procaine penicillin, in cattle, poultry, and pigs was first shown to have a growth-promoting impact in the mid-1950s. In 1951, the FDA first approved the use of antibiotics as an addition in animal feed. Antibiotic dose recommendations as growth promoters in animal feed have increased from 10 to 20 g/ton in the 1950s to 30 to 110 g/ton now. The United States leads the world in the usage of antibiotics as feed additives, adding 86 g of antibiotics per tonne of animal feed. China follows with 74 g of antibiotics per tonne of feed, which is 30 and 12%, respectively, more than the average use of 66 g of antibiotic per ton of feed worldwide.

Role of Antibiotics in Poultry Industry

The antibiotics used in the chicken industry can be divided into three categories: growth promoters, prophylactic antibiotics and therapeutic antibiotics. In the poultry industry, veterinarians use antibiotics to improve growth, feed efficiency, and lower disease. The efficient raising of chickens made possible using antibiotics has allowed consumers to affordably acquire premium meat and eggs. Because antibiotic use lowers the incidence of sickness, it has also improved the health and wellbeing of chickens. The mid-1950s saw the prescription of antimicrobial medicines for the goal of promoting growth in agricultural animals. Since then, the chicken industry has widely used supplementary feeds containing subtherapeutic dosages of tetracycline, chloramphenicol, and procaine penicillin to encourage growth and egg production. Several ionophores, tylosin, avoparcin, and virginiamycin have also been employed as growth promoters. Antibiotics may stimulate growth through their antimicrobial activity against pathogens and dangerous bacteria, even though the precise processes by which they do so are yet unknown. Antimicrobial drugs have been proposed to prevent intestinal bacterial growth, thus shielding nutrients from bacterial degradation.

Antibiotics for Both Preventative and Therapeutic Use

The most used medications in the poultry business are antibiotics, which are naturally occurring, semi-synthetic, or synthetic substances with antibacterial action. The most widely used antibiotics are: tetracycline, gentamicin, neomycin, tylosine, erythromycin, virginiamycin, ceftiofur, and bacitracin. These drugs are typically helpful in reducing and preventing infections related to necrotic enteritis and respiratory diseases; gastroenteritis, skin, or soft tissue infections are treated with fluoroquinolones and/or quinolone compounds; sulphonamide compounds are used as preventive and chemotherapeutic agents against pullorum disease, fowl typhoid, coryza, and pullorum disease; coccidiosis is treated with piperazine, oxytetracycline, amoxicillin, amprolium, cipro floxacillin, and sulfa drugs. To prevent and treat coccidiosis, numerous anticoccidial medications (such as nicarbazin, salinomycin, sulphonamides, clopidol, amprolium, etc.) and vaccines (made from non-attenuated or attenuated oocysts of coccidia strains) are frequently used as antidotes in chicken feed.

Mechanism of Action of AGPs (antibiotic growth promoters)

The precise method by which antibiotics function as growth-promoting drugs is still unknown, although it is thought to be connected to AGP interactions with the intestinal microbial population. There are four main theories explaining the growth improvement linked with AGP. These include preventing endemic infections from spreading in the first place, reducing the number of metabolites produced by microorganisms that could stunt growth, decreasing the amount of nutrients that are absorbed by gut-related microbes, and improving the animal's ability to absorb and use nutrients due to the intestinal wall's thinning. Nonetheless, by reducing the gut microbiota's growth-suppressive actions, the AGPs enhance bird growth. Contrary to earlier theories that suggested AGPs interacted directly with gut microbes, the anti-inflammatory impact of these medicines has been demonstrated. The mechanism suggests that intestinal inflammatory cells impede the production and release of catabolic mediating molecules. The microbiota is altered because of the intestinal wall's subsequent change in condition. Nevertheless, further research is needed to determine the precise mechanism by which antibiotics promote growth.

Antibiotic Residues

Even though everyone involved benefits from these uses, however, consumers believe that edible fowl tissues contain dangerously high levels of drug residues. On the other hand, the overuse of antibiotics might contribute to the emergence of resistance by means of mechanisms such as the build-up of antibiotic residues in the human food chain. The use of antibiotics in food animals poses a significant risk to humans due to antibiotic resistance development among bacteria. Antibiotic use is linked to the formation of resistant germs in animals, which then spread to humans via food, the environment, and direct contact with the infected meat. Antimicrobial chemical residues are also discovered in animal-derived foods because of their incorrect or excessive use. These residues are also known to get to humans via food and the environment.

Significance for Consumer Health

Despite the restrictions, a lot of layers and broiler chickens receive overdoses or improper dosages of antibiotic medications for preventative, therapeutic, and non-therapeutic uses throughout their lives. These medications would not be hazardous if they were not absorbed or metabolized by the animal, but that is not always the case. As a result, toxic medication residues often build up in different amounts in the animal parts that humans consume. Parent and derivative chemicals, such as metabolites, conjugates and leftovers bound to macromolecules, make up most of these residues. Consuming organs and tissues (meat, offal, eggs, etc.) that have medication remains beyond safe maximum residual levels (MRLs) can lead to several health risks and vulnerabilities that are directly linked to the development of hypersensitivity or allergic reactions, cutaneous eruptions, dermatitis, alteration of intestinal microflora, etc.

In addition to other negative effects like immunopathological effects, autoimmunity, carcinogenicity (oxytetracycline), mutagenicity, nephropathy (gentamicin), hepatotoxicity, reproductive disorders, bone marrow toxicity, and allergy (penicillin), may increase the risk of food-borne infection with antibiotic-resistant pathogenic bacteria. Due to the extremely low amounts of residues in food, toxic effects are unlikely. This issue is more important as many chicken products on the market are not subjected to an antibiotic residue analysis.

The Principal Methods for Antibiotic Residue Detection

There are two ways used to identify antibiotic residues in chicken and its products: the screening approach and the confirmatory method. The first approach is universally qualitative or semiquantitative, which sets it apart from the other two. On the other hand, the latter guarantees a very accurate identification of the kind and amount of residue under investigation.

Screening Method

In essence, all screening techniques are either immunological or microbiological. The so-called "four plates" method is the most well-known and ancient microbiological technique. *Bacillus subtilis* and *Micrococcus luteus* growth inhibition is achieved by this method. The absence of bacterial colonies in the inhibitory zones surrounding the sample deposit locations suggests the possible presence of antibiotics. Examining the prevalence of antibiotic residues in various meats, fish, and eggs is a common usage for this technique. Immunological techniques, such as enzyme-linked immunosorbent assay, fluor immunoassay, and time-resolved fluor immunoassay, are simpler, more affordable, and have higher specificity and sensitivity than microbiological techniques.

Confirmatory Methods

In essence, confirmatory techniques involve chromatographic techniques—primarily liquid chromatography coupled to ultraviolet (UV) or mass spectrometry. Nevertheless, it has also been demonstrated that capillary electrophoresis (CE), surface-enhanced Raman spectroscopy, CE-laser-induced fluorescence, and high-performance liquid chromatography (HPLC) with spectroscopic HPLC-photodiode array detector or spectroscopic HPLC-fluorometric detection (HPLC-RF) are efficient methods for detecting antibiotic residues. The primary benefit of confirmatory procedures is their high specificity; nevertheless, they come at a cost, take a lot of time, and need staff and a suitable laboratory.

National and International Initiatives Addressing Antibiotic Resistance

To control and monitor the use of antibiotics in food animals and the ensuing development of antibiotic resistance, the World Health Organisation (WHO), Food and Agricultural Organisation (FAO), World Organisation for Animal Health (OIE), European Union (EU), European Centre for Disease Prevention and Control (ECDC), and governments worldwide are dedicated to creating guidelines and policies. The WHO has approved the "One Health Approach" as a means of addressing this issue on a worldwide scale through the "Tripartite Alliance," an alliance that consists of the WHO, FAO, and OIE. The World Health Organisation (WHO) released the "Global Action Plan (GAP) on antimicrobial resistance" in collaboration with its three partners in 2015. The GAP focuses on several tactics, such as enhancing hygiene, sanitation, and cleanliness; increasing awareness of antimicrobial resistance; fortifying surveillance; encouraging research; lowering the incidence of infections; and optimising the use of antibiotics in conjunction with enhanced treatments. It also offers strategic recommendations for reducing the danger of zoonosis and related hazards related to animal food safety. The WHO has also placed a value on antibiotics and antimicrobials in relation to human treatment, limited the use of these drugs in animals raised for food, and set aside specific drug classes exclusively for human use. Additionally, the FAO has started implementing the WHO's GAP in the animal food and agriculture sectors through the "AMR Strategy." The adoption of veterinary laws and rules allowing the use of "Veterinary Critically Important Antimicrobial Agents, Veterinary Highly Important Antimicrobial Agents, and Veterinary Important Antimicrobial Agents" in court has been emphasised by the OIE.

India, one of the nations most impacted by AMR, is currently taking the necessary actions to address the growing issue of drug resistance by using antibiotics for both human and animal usage under the law. The Bureau of Indian Standards of Poultry Feed advised against using antimicrobials or antibiotics with systemic action as feed additives to boost antibiotic growth in 2007. The Food Safety and Standard Authority of India published regulations on antibiotic residues, toxins, and other pollutants in various food products, including meat and meat products, in December 2018. 2012. The National Policy for Containment of Antimicrobial Resistance was published by the Ministry of Health and Family Welfare.

Methods for Mitigating Antibiotic Residues in Food

The issue of antibiotic residues should be known to both individuals and legal organisations. Utilising probiotics and compounds produced from plants as antibiotic substitutes may be advantageous. It is important to reduce the use of unneeded antibiotics in animals and to take preventative antibiotic use into consideration. The use of antibiotics in animals and the amount of residue they can leave in food should be regulated by legislation in every nation. The use of antibiotics to maintain the health of livestock was outlawed by the EU in 2006. Meat and meat products include traces of carcinogenic substances and/or their genotoxic metabolites in the United States. FDA restrictions have successfully stopped food-borne allergens, toxins, and carcinogens from originating from animal drugs. Despite this, the FDA only authorises novel animal medications under certain conditions: (I) the medication must be taken in small doses; (ii) it cannot cause cancer; and (iii) no residues from the medication may be found in the tissues or products of the animals after an appropriate period has passed. The FDA forbids the use of sulphonamides, fluoroquinolones, furazolidone, nitrofurazone, and chloramphenicol in nursing animals. Veterinarians should also refrain from using medications irrationally. Antibiotic residues can be rendered inactive using cooking and freezing techniques. Animal meals that have been heated may inactivate antibiotics.

Numerous studies have shown that temperature affects the rate at which β-lactams, quinolones, sulphonamides, macrolides, tetracyclines, and aminoglycosides degrade, and that heating for longer periods of time accelerates this process. Inactivating antibiotics may be aided by resin, UV light, and activated charcoal. To detect antibiotic residues in animal products, inexpensive and straightforward field testing could be created, and ethno-veterinary procedures could be encouraged.

Conclusions

To accommodate the growing demand for meat, poultry farms worldwide are using antibiotics on a big scale. Due to various laws, rules, and oversight procedures implemented by governing bodies, there is a great deal of variation in the kinds of antibiotics prescribed globally. Although there are regulations in place in some nations restricting the use of antibiotics on animals, their application is not routinely inspected. Numerous investigations showed that chicken meat had antibiotic levels beyond the maximum residue limits, a sign of the overuse of antibiotics in some nations. Extended use of antibiotics tends to reduce the population of susceptible bacteria, leading to a high proportion of resistant bacterial strains in the microbiome. There have been numerous reports of these resistant strains being transferred to people. Through genetic transfer, these strains may impart their virulence to the human microbiome. If or when certain bacterial strains produce infection, treating them can be challenging. Certain researches suggest that cooking procedures could lower the amounts of antibiotic residue. It does not, however, provide total removal of antibiotic residues from foods, hence it might not be considered a substitute for residue removal. Furthermore, antibiotics that are deemed essential by various regulatory bodies, such as the FDA and the World Health Organisation, need not to be used agriculture.

4

Phyto-biotics Effective Strategy to Mitigate Antimicrobial Resistance in Poultry-Linked Foodborne Zoonoses

Reshma M.M. and Aswathi P.B.

Department of Poultry Science, College of Veterinary and Animal Sciences Pookode, Kerala Veterinary and Animal Sciences University, Kerala

The poultry industry in India is experiencing rapid growth, with meat production and egg production increasing by 5.13% and 6.77%, respectively, in 2022-2023 compared to the previous year (BAHS, 2023). Numerous factors and challenges impact poultry production on a global scale, such as intense international competition, evolving consumer attitudes toward food safety, animal welfare, and environmental conservation. Poultry commonly harbor infectious diseases that can also affect humans, with many of these zoonotic diseases having reservoirs in mammalian species other than humans, adding complexity to their management. Foodborne illnesses, primarily attributed to *Salmonella* serovars and *Campylobacter* spp., represent the predominant bacterial agents responsible for human foodborne diseases associated with poultry. There are suggestions that *Escherichia coli* originating from poultry could lead to human illness, thereby necessitating *E. coli* to be regarded as a potential foodborne pathogen. Furthermore, the emergence of antibiotic-resistant bacteria will persist as a threat to public health (Hafez and Hauck, 2023). Hence, it is imperative to promptly discover and implement innovative approaches to address antibiotic resistance, utilizing a range of strategies such as probiotics, prebiotics, phytobiotics and others (Helmy *et al.*, 2023).

Foodborne Zoonoses Linked to Poultry

Each year, 600 million instances of foodborne illnesses and 4,20,000 fatalities occur globally as a result of contaminated food. 7.69 per cent of the world's

7.8 billion inhabitants suffer from food-borne illnesses each year and 7.5 per cent of all fatalities worldwide each year (56 million) are attributable to these infections (Lee and Yoon, 2021). The main zoonotic bacterial pathogens that cause food-borne disease and mortality worldwide linked to consumption of tainted animal products are *S. aureus*, *Salmonella* species, *Campylobacter* species, *L. monocytogenes* and *E. coli* (Abebe *et al.*, 2020).

Campylobacteriosis stands as the most frequently reported gastroenteritic illness transmitted through food and imposes a significant health burden in developed nations. Human infection is predominantly attributed to the zoonotic pathogen *Campylobacter jejuni.* Given its pervasive presence in the environment, the epidemiology of *Campylobacter* remains inadequately elucidated. Nonetheless, there is consensus that chickens serve as a natural reservoir for *Campylobacter jejuni* and other *Campylobacter* species, with colonized broiler chicks identified as the primary means of transmitting this pathogen to humans (Hermans *et al.,* 2012). As per the 2020 EFSA Scientific Opinion, a significant contamination detected in specific categories of fresh meat underscores the pivotal role of these products in the epidemiology of campylobacteriosis, whether through direct handling or cross-contamination with other foods. Across broilers, turkeys, and other fresh meat, the overall percentages of *Campylobacter*-positive samples were notably high, at 30.1%, 21%, and 25.1%, respectively (EFSA , 2021). In terms of *Campylobacter* contamination levels in chicken meat, data from 2018 indicate that almost 20% of carcasses tested positive for *Campylobacter* at slaughter, while about 9% of chicken breast samples were positive at retail (Williams *et al.*, 2021).

Salmonella infections originating from food and animals remain a persistent threat to public health on a global scale (Ramatla *et al.*, 2019). Non-typhoidal salmonellosis (NTS) arises from various *Salmonella* serovars apart from Typhi, Sendai, and Paratyphi (Dróżdż *et al.*, 2021). Roughly 1% of cases of acute gastroenteritis among children under five years old in Kolkata, India, were attributed to non-typhoidal *Salmonella* (NTS), with *S.* Worthington (33%), *S.* Enteritidis (13%), and *S.* Typhimurium (12%) serovars being the most prevalent (Jain *et al.*, 2020). According to estimates, 86 per cent of all NTS infections in the globe are food-borne. A lot of human epidemics have been linked to eggs and chicken meat (Ford *et al.*, 2018). A considerable proportion of food-borne infections (17.9 per cent) are linked to chicken, and *S.enterica* was responsible for 19 per cent of those cases (O'Bryan *et al.*, 2022). The most prevalent serotypes found in food items are *S.* Typhimurium, *S.*Enteritidis and *S.*Newport, which cause 50 per cent of salmonellosis (Dar *et al.*, 2017). One of the primary causes of non-typhoidal salmonellosis is eating chicken products (Shivaprasad, 2013).The ability to endure and progress through the many stages of poultry production determines its presence in the food sector (Vinueza-Burgos *et al.*, 2019).

Avian pathogenic *Escherichia coli* (APEC), categorized as an extra-intestinal pathogenic *E. coli* (ExPEC), induces a range of localized and systemic infections in various avian species such as chickens, turkeys, ducks, and numerous other birds. Numerous studies have indicated that APEC could serve as a potential zoonotic pathogen transmitted through food, in addition to being a potential source or reservoir of extra-intestinal infections in humans. This is primarily attributed to its genetic resemblance to human ExPECs, the presence of virulence genes common to or defining human ExPECs, and its capability to induce urinary tract infections (UTIs) and meningitis in rodent models, similar to uropathogenic *E. coli* (UPEC) and neonatal meningitis-causing *E. coli* (NMEC) (Kathayat *et al.*, 2021).

The Rise of Antimicrobial Resistance Among Zoonotic Pathogens in Poultry Products

Antimicrobial resistance (AMR) occurs when bacteria, viruses, fungi, and parasites can thrive despite previous susceptibility to drugs. The Centers for Disease Control and Prevention (CDC) approximates that antibiotic resistance leads to a $20 billion rise in direct healthcare costs annually in the United States, not including an estimated $35 billion in productivity losses (Dadgostar, 2019). Multiple classes of antimicrobial drugs are employed in both food-producing and companion animals, mirroring their usage in human health. Resistance emerging in one setting can undermine the effectiveness of drugs utilized in other environments (McDermott *et al.*, 2018). The primary contributors to antimicrobial resistance (AMR) include the improper utilization of antimicrobials in the feed and poultry sectors, widespread administration in patients with diverse medical conditions, gene transfer, mutation, and selective pressure. Inadequate management of meat and its products in slaughterhouses also significantly contributes to the spread and occurrence of new multidrug-resistant (MDR) strains (Salam *et al.*, 2023).

A study conducted by Hull *et al.* (2021) reported that total 90.4% (489 out of 541) of Campylobacter isolates were found to possess antimicrobial resistance (AMR) genes. Among them, 43% (233 out of 541) harbored genes conferring resistance to three or more classes of antibiotics, indicating molecular multidrug resistance. The prevalence of AMR genes was highest against tetracyclines (64.3%), beta-lactams (63.6%), aminoglycosides (38.6%), macrolides (34.8%), quinolones (24.4%), lincosamides (13.5%), and streptothricins (5%).

The significant levels of antimicrobial resistance observed in Campylobacter isolated from chicken carcasses during 2009-2018 underscore the urgent need to minimize antimicrobial usage in poultry treatment. Additionally, there is a call for the adoption of targeted control measures aimed at reducing campylobacter contamination levels on chicken carcasses (Wieczorek *et al.*, 2020). Globally, the median prevalence of Salmonella in broiler chickens stands at 40.5%, with corresponding figures of 30% in raw chicken meat and 40.5% in eggs and egg-laying hens. Furthermore, there is an elevated occurrence of multidrug-resistant (MDR) isolates originating from poultry farms (91.1%) and raw chicken meat obtained from processing plants and markets (97.8%) worldwide. Notably, the most pronounced levels of antibiotic resistance within the poultry production chain were observed for nalidixic acid and ampicillin. Likewise, multidrug-resistant (MDR) *E. coli* isolates were commonly found among poultry workers, poultry itself, and the poultry farm/live bird market (LBM) environment. These isolates exhibited a high prevalence of resistance, particularly against tetracycline (92.7%), trimethoprim/sulfamethoxazole (84.5%), streptomycin (79.1%), and ampicillin (80%) (Aworh *et al.*, 2021). In 2019, the six primary pathogens contributing to deaths linked to resistance were *Escherichia coli*, *Staphylococcus aureus*, *Klebsiella pneumoniae*, *Streptococcus pneumoniae*, *Acinetobacter baumannii* and *Pseudomonas aeruginosa*. These pathogens were accountable for an estimated 929,000 deaths directly attributed to antimicrobial resistance (AMR) and approximately 3.57 million deaths associated with AMR (Murray *et al.*, 2022).

Quantitatively, the global consumption of antimicrobial drugs in livestock was approximately 63,151 tonnes in 2010. Projections indicate a 67% surge by 2030, reaching around 105,500 tonnes, driven by the escalating demand for livestock products in middle-income nations among the human population (Van Boeckel *et al.*, 2015). According to the World Bank, in the most favorable scenario with minimal impact from antimicrobial resistance (AMR), the global gross domestic product (GDP) is projected to decrease by 1.1% by 2050. In the worst-case scenario, this reduction could reach 3.8%. This equates to an annual deficit of $3.4 trillion by 2030 (World Bank, 2017).

Strategies for Addressing Antimicrobial Resistance

The World Health Assembly has endorsed five strategic action plans to tackle AMR. These include: (1) enhancing awareness and comprehension of antimicrobial resistance; (2) strengthening knowledge through surveillance and research to combat infections via control measures; (3) deploying efficient sanitation, hygiene, and infection prevention measures; (4) optimising the usage of antimicrobials in both human and animal health; and (5) promoting sustainable investment in new medicines, diagnostic tools, and vaccines (WHO, 2015). The adoption of antibiotic alternatives is among the interventions aimed at combating antimicrobial resistance. Recent research suggests that plants represent untapped reservoirs of potential antimicrobial agents, with compounds like polyphenolics, alkaloids, and various plant extracts gaining attention for their therapeutic properties (Othman *et al.*, 2019). Phytobiotics, derived from plants or plant extracts, are employed to enhance the health and productivity of various animal species, including poultry. This encompasses the utilization of both herbs (non-woody and non-perennial plants) and spices (highly aromatic and flavorful herbs) (Kuralkar and Kuralkar, 2021).

Effects of Dietary Supplementation of Phytobiotics as a Strategy to Control foodborne Zoonoses Linked to Poultry

Salmonella Infection

Garlic extract exhibited *in vitro* inhibition of *S.* Typhimurium, *S.* Papuana, *S.* Inganda, *S.* Kentucky, *S.* Enteritidis, *S.* Heidelberg, *S.* Molade, *S.* Tamale, *S.* Labadi (Minimum inhibitory concentration ranging from 40–100 mg/mL), accompanied by reduced mortality and enhanced body weight observed in chickens supplemented challenged with *S.* Typhimurium (Salem *et al.*, 2017). The addition of purified capsaicin in broilers resulted in a decrease in *S.* Enteritidis colonization in the liver/spleen and ceca. Incorporating 5 ppm of capsaicin led to reduced *S.* Enteritidis colonization in the ceca and a decrease in cecal lamina propria thickness (Orndoff *et al.*, 2005). A phytogenic feed additive containing essential oils (carvacrol, thymol, and cinnamic aldehyde) reduced the total bacterial count by 1% when included in the broiler feed. Additionally, the inclusion of the feed additive resulted in increased total erythrocyte counts and hemoglobin content, accompanied by a decrease in lymphocyte counts (Reis *et al.*, 2018). Administering a commercial phytobiotic supplement composed of a blend of essential oils (containing garlic, lemon, thyme, and eucalyptus), upregulated the genes AvBD10, IL6, IL8L2, CASP6, and IRF7 on the first day post-infection. However, their expression decreased in the infected birds by day 23 (Laptev *et al.*, 2019). Supplementing broilers with phytobiotics containing sanguinarine and oregano enhanced growth performance and gut health by mitigating the adverse effects of *S.* Typhimurium infection (Aljumaah *et al.*, 2020).

Campylobacter Infection

Various essential oils, polyphenols, and terpenoid compounds were evaluated against C. jejuni, with notable potency observed in essential oils and terpenoid compounds (Kurekci *et al.*, 2013). In their study, Arsi *et al.* (2014) reported positive outcomes with the application of 0.25% and 2% thymol, as well as 1% carvacrol, and a combination of 0.5% thymol and carvacrol. Encapsulated phenolic-rich fraction (PRF) derived from Ferula gummosa leaves has the potential to enhance growth parameters, liver enzymes, and lipid peroxidation. It also improves the morphometric parameters of the ileum and inhibits the population of *C. jejuni* in the ileum of mice challenged with *C. jejuni* infection (Kamelan *et al.*, 2022). Chicken breast fillets treated with a combination of 5 ml of turmeric, lemon, and green tea extracts were capable of eliminating all *C.* jejuni and *S.* Enteritidis within 12 hours of incubation. Conversely, using single extracts alone was ineffective in achieving the same outcome, as demonstrated in the study (Murali *et al.*, 2012).

Conclusion

The utilisation of phytobiotics in animals presents a promising avenue for combating foodborne pathogens linked to poultry in the context of antimicrobial resistance. Through the exploration of plant-derived compounds and extracts, phytobiotics offer a natural and potentially effective alternative to traditional antimicrobial agents. While research continues to uncover the specific mechanisms and optimal formulations of phytobiotics, evidence suggests their ability to inhibit the growth and virulence of foodborne pathogens, even in the face of antimicrobial resistance. Moving forward, further investigation and implementation of phytobiotics in food production and processing may contribute significantly to mitigating the spread of antimicrobial resistance and enhancing food safety for consumers worldwide.

References

Abebe, E., Gugsa, G. and Ahmed, M. 2020. Review on major food-borne zoonotic bacterial pathogens. J. Trop. Med. 2020: 1-19

Aljumaah, M.R., Alkhulaifi, M.M., Aljumaah, R.S., Abudabos, A.M., Abdullatif, A.A., Suliman, G.M., Mu'ath, Q. and Stanley, D., 2020. Influence of sanguinarine-based phytobiotic supplementation on post necrotic enteritis challenge recovery. Heliyon, 6(11).

Arsi, K., Donoghue, A.M., Venkitanarayanan, K., Kollanoor-Johny, A., Fanatico, A.C., Blore, P.J. and Donoghue, D.J., 2014. The efficacy of the natural plant extracts, thymol and carvacrol against C ampylobacter colonization in broiler chickens. Journal of Food Safety, 34(4), pp.321-325.

Aworh, M.K., Kwaga, J.K., Hendriksen, R.S., Okolocha, E.C. and Thakur, S., 2021. Genetic relatedness of multidrug resistant Escherichia coli isolated from humans, chickens and poultry environments. Antimicrobial Resistance & Infection Control, 10, pp.1-13.

Bank, W., 2017. Drug-resistant infections: a threat to our economic future. World Bank.

Dadgostar, P. 2019. Antimicrobial resistance: implications and costs. Infect. Drug Resist. 12: 3903-3910.

Dar, M.A., Ahmad, S.M., Bhat, S.A., Ahmed, R., Urwat, U., Mumtaz, P.T., Bhat, S.A., Dar, T.A., Shah, R.A. and Ganai, N.A. 2017. Salmonella Typhimurium in poultry: a review. World's Poult. Sci. J. 73: 345-354.

Dróżdż, M., Małaszczuk, M., Paluch, E. and Pawlak, A., 2021. Zoonotic potential and prevalence of Salmonella serovars isolated from pets. Infection Ecology & Epidemiology, 11(1), p.1975530.

European Food Safety Authority and European Centre for Disease Prevention and Control, 2021. The European Union one health 2020 zoonoses report. EFSA Journal, 19(12), p.e06971.

Ford, L., Moffatt, C.R., Fearnley, E., Miller, M., Gregory, J., Sloan-Gardner, T.S., Polkinghorne, B.G., Bell, R., Franklin, N., Williamson, D.A. and Glass, K. 2018. The epidemiology of Salmonella enterica outbreaks in Australia, 2001–2016. Front. Sustain. Food Syst. 2: 86.

Hafez, H.M. and Hauck, R., 2023. Zoonoses Transmitted by Poultry: Risks Related to Poultry Rearing and Eating Poultry Products. In Zoonoses: Infections Affecting Humans and Animals (pp. 207-230). Cham: Springer International Publishing.

Helmy, Y.A., Taha-Abdelaziz, K., Hawwas, H.A.E.H., Ghosh, S., AlKafaas, S.S., Moawad, M.M., Saied, E.M., Kassem, I.I. and Mawad, A.M., 2023. Antimicrobial Resistance and Recent Alternatives to Antibiotics for the Control of Bacterial Pathogens with an Emphasis on Foodborne Pathogens. Antibiotics, 12(2), p.274.

Hermans, D., Pasmans, F., Messens, W., Martel, A., Van Immerseel, F., Rasschaert, G., Heyndrickx, M., Van Deun, K. and Haesebrouck, F., 2012. Poultry as a host for the zoonotic pathogen Campylobacter jejuni. Vector-Borne and Zoonotic Diseases, 12(2), pp.89-98.

Hull, D.M., Harrell, E., van Vliet, A.H., Correa, M. and Thakur, S., 2021. Antimicrobial resistance and interspecies gene transfer in Campylobacter coli and Campylobacter jejuni isolated from food animals, poultry processing, and retail meat in North Carolina, 2018–2019. PLoS One, 16(2), p.e0246571.

Jain, P., Chowdhury, G., Samajpati, S., Basak, S., Ganai, A., Samanta, S., Okamoto, K., Mukhopadhyay, A.K. and Dutta, S., 2020. Characterization of non-typhoidal Salmonella isolates from children with acute gastroenteritis, Kolkata, India, during 2000–2016. Brazilian Journal of Microbiology, 51, pp.613-627.

Kamelan Kafi, M., Bolvari, N.E., Mohammad Pour, S., Moghadam, S.K., Shafaei, N., Karimi, E. and Oskoueian, E., 2022. Encapsulated phenolic compounds from Ferula gummosa leaf: A potential phytobiotic against Campylobacter jejuni infection. Journal of Food Processing and Preservation, 46(8), p.e16802.

Kathayat, D., Lokesh, D., Ranjit, S. and Rajashekara, G., 2021. Avian pathogenic Escherichia coli (APEC): an overview of virulence and pathogenesis factors, zoonotic potential, and control strategies. Pathogens, 10(4), p.467.

Kuralkar, P. and Kuralkar, S.V., 2021. Role of herbal products in animal production–An updated review. Journal of Ethnopharmacology, 278, p.114246.

Kurekci, C., Padmanabha, J., Bishop-Hurley, S.L., Hassan, E., Al Jassim, R.A. and McSweeney, C.S., 2013. Antimicrobial activity of essential oils and five terpenoid compounds against Campylobacter jejuni in pure and mixed culture experiments. International journal of food microbiology, 166(3), pp.450-457.

Laptev, G.Y., Filippova, V.A., Kochish, I.I., Yildirim, E.A., Ilina, L.A., Dubrovin, A.V., Brazhnik, E.A., Novikova, N.I., Novikova, O.B., Dmitrieva, M.E. and Smolensky, V.I., 2019. Examination of the expression of immunity genes and bacterial profiles in the caecum of growing chickens infected with Salmonella Enteritidis and fed a phytobiotic. Animals, 9(9), p.615.

McDermott, P.F., Tyson, G.H., Kabera, C., Chen, Y., Li, C., Folster, J.P., Ayers, S.L., Lam, C., Tate, H.P. and Zhao, S. 2016. Whole-genome sequencing for detecting antimicrobial resistance in nontyphoidal Salmonella. Antimicrob. Agents Chemother. 60: 5515-5520.

Murali, N., Kumar-Phillips, G.S., Rath, N.C., Marcy, J. and Slavik, M.F., 2012. Effect of marinating chicken meat with lemon, green tea and turmeric against foodborne bacterial pathogens. International Journal of Poultry Science, 11(5), p.326.

Murray, C.J., Ikuta, K.S., Sharara, F., Swetschinski, L., Aguilar, G.R., Gray, A., Han, C., Bisignano, C., Rao, P., Wool, E. and Johnson, S.C., 2022. Global burden of bacterial antimicrobial resistance in 2019: a systematic analysis. The Lancet, 399(10325), pp.629-655.

Orndorff, B.W., Novak, C.L., Pierson, F.W., Caldwell, D.J. and McElroy, A.P., 2005. Comparison of prophylactic or therapeutic dietary administration of capsaicin for reduction of Salmonella in broiler chickens. Avian Diseases, 49(4), pp.527-533.

Othman, L., Sleiman, A. and Abdel-Massih, R.M., 2019. Antimicrobial activity of polyphenols and alkaloids in middle eastern plants. Frontiers in Microbiology, 10, p.911.

O'Bryan, C.A., Ricke, S.C. and Marcy, J.A. 2022. Public health impact of Salmonella spp. on raw poultry: current concepts and future prospects in the United States. Food Control. 132: 108539.

Ramatla, T., Taioe, M.O., Thekisoe, O.M. and Syakalima, M., 2019. Confirmation of antimicrobial resistance by using resistance genes of isolated Salmonella spp. in chicken houses of North West, South Africa. World's Veterinary Journal, 9(3), pp.158-165.

Reis, J.H., Gebert, R.R., Barreta, M., Baldissera, M.D., Dos Santos, I.D., Wagner, R., Campigotto, G., Jaguezeski, A.M., Gris, A., de Lima, J.L. and Mendes, R.E., 2018. Effects of phytogenic feed additive based on thymol, carvacrol and cinnamic aldehyde on body weight, blood parameters and environmental bacteria in broilers chickens. Microbial pathogenesis, 125, pp.168-176.

Salam, M.A., Al-Amin, M.Y., Salam, M.T., Pawar, J.S., Akhter, N., Rabaan, A.A. and Alqumber, M.A. 2023. Antimicrobial Resistance: A Growing Serious Threat for Global Public Health. Healthc. 11: 1946.

Salem, W.M., El-Hamed, D.M.S., Sayed, W.F. and Elamary, R.B., 2017. Alterations in virulence and antibiotic resistant genes of multidrug-resistant Salmonella serovars isolated from poultry: The bactericidal efficacy of Allium sativum. Microbial pathogenesis, 108, pp.91-100.

Shivaprasad, H.L. 2013. Salmonella infections in the domestic fowl. In: Methner, U. and Barrow, P.A.Salmonella in domestic animals. CABI, Wallingford UK, pp. 162-192.

Van Boeckel, T.P., Brower, C., Gilbert, M., Grenfell, B.T., Levin, S.A., Robinson, T.P., Teillant, A. and Laxminarayan, R., 2015. Global trends in antimicrobial use in food animals. Proceedings of the National Academy of Sciences, 112(18), pp.5649-5654.

Vinueza-Burgos, C., Baquero, M., Medina, J. and De Zutter, L. 2019. Occurrence, genotypes and antimicrobial susceptibility of Salmonella collected from the broiler production chain within an integrated poultry company. Int. J. Food Microbiol.299: 1-7.

WHO. Global Action Plan on Antibiotic Resistance. Available online: https://www.emro.who.int/health-topics/drug-resistance/global-action-plan.html (accessed on 05 February 2024).

Wieczorek, K., Bocian, Ł. and Osek, J., 2020. Prevalence and antimicrobial resistance of Campylobacter isolated from carcasses of chickens slaughtered in Poland–a retrospective study. Food control, 112, p.107159.

Williams, M.S., Ebel, E.D. and Nyirabahizi, E., 2021. Comparative history of Campylobacter contamination on chicken meat and campylobacteriosis cases in the United States: 1994–2018. International Journal of Food Microbiology, 342, p.109075.

5

Turmeric, Amla and Giloy Alternatives to Antibiotic Growth Promoter in Broiler Farming

Gurram Srinivas[1], Sushmasri Kandanulu[2], Swathi Bora[3] M. Hanumanth Rao[4], Sai Reddy[5], Divya Begari[6]

[1&4]Poultry Research Station
[2]NDRI, Karnal
[3]Department of Veterinary Pathology
[5]Animal Husbandry Polytechnic- Mamnoor
[6]ICAR -DPR
P.V. Narsimha Rao Telangana Veterinary University, Rajendranagar, Hyderabad, Telangana, India

---

Poultry is one of the fastest growing segments of livestock in India. The major growth promoters used in broiler diets in the past were antibiotics, which have been found helpful in improvement of growth performance and feed conversion ratio in poultry (Miles *et al.*, 2006). However, constant supplementation of antibiotic growth promoters (AGP) in poultry feed led to residual effects in poultry products and usage of antibiotics in sub-therapeutic concentrations resulted in development of antibiotic resistant bacteria (Diaz *et al.*, 2015) which represent a public health hazard. Owing to increased health concerns that come with consumption of meat loaded with antibiotic residues, European Union imposed ban on using antibiotics in animal feeds as growth promoters in 2006. Since then, alternatives for AGPs were being evaluated to improve the performance of livestock and poultry (Windisch *et al.*, 2008).

Most of the studies have been done on usage of botanicals which were used in human feed as additives traditionally. The beneficial effects of botanicals and their extracts are related to stimulating digestive enzymes and antioxidants, increasing digestibility, improving gut histology (Jamroz *et al.*, 2003), stabilizing the microbiota and reducing microbial toxins, reduces inflammation and allocation of protein to growth (Kroismayr *et al.*, 2008). The beneficial effects of botanicals are linked to the phytochemical constituents present in them like terpenoids, phenolics, flavonoids, glycosides and alkaloids (Wenk, 2006). Anew plants like turmeric, amla and giloy extracts either individually or in combination are in use as alternative to AGPs.

Curcuma longa commonly known as turmeric, contains numerous bioactive compounds which possess different pharmacological activities such as antioxidant property, property of stimulating pancreatic enzymes, immune modulating (Lee *et al.*, 2013), anti-inflammatory, anti-microbial, anti-cancer (Gera *et al.*, 2017), hypo-cholesterolemic, hypo lipemic and enhancing phagocytic activity (Chakraborty *et al.*, 2011).

Amla scientifically called *Emblica officinalis* / *Phyllanthus emblica* belongs to the family *Euphorbiaceae*, commonly called as Indian gooseberry is rich in vitamin C (478.56 mg/100 mL) i.e. it contains more vitamin C than oranges, lemons and tangerines (Jain and Khurdiya, 2004). It has innumerable health benefits some of them include antioxidant, immunomodulatory, cytoprotective, gastroprotective, hepatoprotective, cardioprotective, anti-hyperlipidemic, anticancer and anti-ulcer properties (Khan, 2009). Amla contains phytochemicals like tannins, phenolics, amino acids, alkaloids, flavonoids, carbohydrates and high quantity of linoleic acid (Arora *et al.*, 2011).

Tinospora cordifolia belongs to Menispermaceae family is one of the three amrit plants commonly called as giloy and guduchi. The name guduchi is derived from Sanskrit, meaning imperishable. Giloy contains various phytonutrients such as, alkaloids, glycosides, lactones, steroids, polysaccharides and aliphatic compounds which exhibit various sanative properties viz. anti-inflammatory, immunomodulatory (Raghu *et al.*, 2009), cognition, antineoplastic, hypoglycemic, hypolipemic (Kumar, 2015), antioxidant, anti-allergic, antituberculosis, anti-osteoporotic, gastrointestinal and hepatoprotection properties (Dwivedi and Enespa, 2016).

Turmeric

Turmeric (*Curcuma longa*) is a rhizomatous herbaceous perennial plant which is a chief source of curcumin and a wide variety of bio active compounds like polyphenols, sesquiterpenes, diterpenes, triterpenoids, sterols and alkaloids. Its major bioactive constituent curcumin possesses various pharmacological properties which include anticancer, antidiabetic, anti-osteoarthritis, antidiarrheal, cardioprotective, anti-oxidative, neuroprotective, hepatoprotective, anti-microbial, reno-protective and anti-inflammatory activities (Iweala *et al.*, 2023).

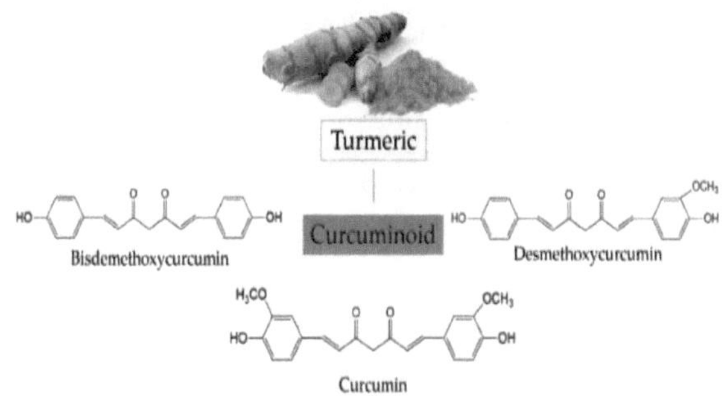

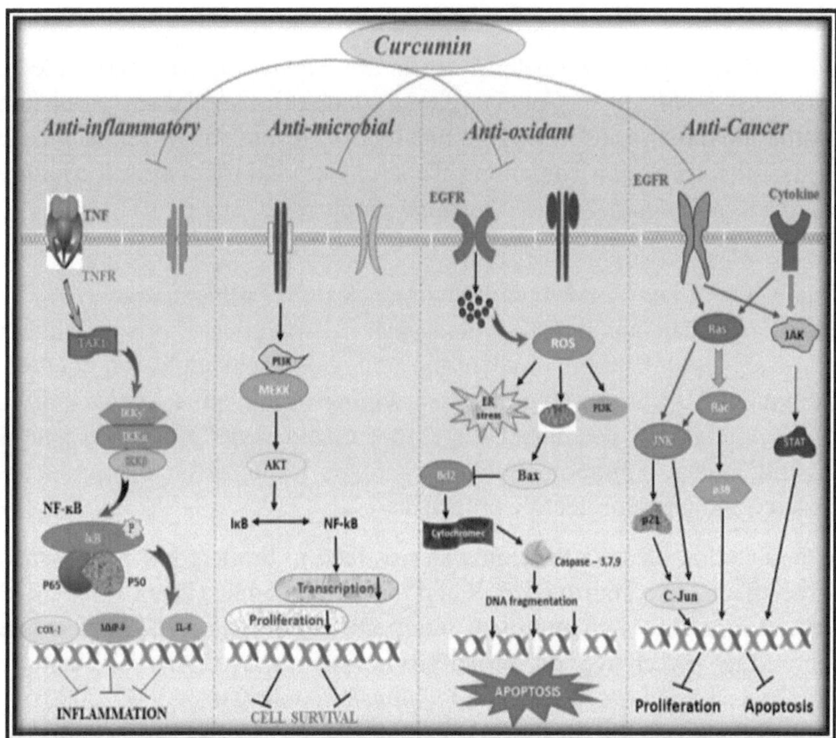

Mechanism of action of curcumin in different biomedical applications Gera *et al.*, 2017

Turmeric possesses appetite stimulant, stomachic and carminative properties (Chakraborty *et al.*, 2011). Curcumin, one of the major phytochemical components of turmeric have been reported to stimulate the digestive enzymes of the pancreas (Platel and Srinivasan, 2004), apoptosis of adipocytes (Sugiharto *et al.*, 2011), inhibition of enzyme responsible for cholesterol synthesis in the liver i.e. hepatic-3-hydroxyl-3-methyglutaryl CoA reductase and it has also been reported that essential oils present in turmeric favors the growth of gut friendly bacteria in chicken (Gul and Bakht, 2015) which improves digestion and absorption of nutrients.

Supplementation of turmeric through diet to broilers has shown many positive effects - some of them include increased feed intake (Chowdhary *et al.*, 2021), improved final live weight gain (Tingare *et al.*, 2023), improved feed conversion ratio (FCR) (Chandra *et al.*, 2019), decreased abdominal fat percentage (Parvin *et al.*, 2021), decrease in total serum cholesterol level (Choudhury *et al.*, 2018), improved serum total protein, albumin and globulin content (Oluwafemi *et al.*, 2021) and increased thigh and breast weights (Hussein, 2013).

Amla

Amla (*Emblica officinalis*) belongs to family *Euphorbiaceae*, also called as *Phyllanthus Emblica,* hatriphala, Amla, Amaliki, Amalakan, Sriphalam, Vayastha and Indian gooseberry. It is mostly used in the form of Triphala which is an herbal formulation containing fruits of *Emblica officinalis*, *Terminalia chebula* and *Terminalia belerica* in equal proportions.

Phyto chemical constituents of amla fruit contains 81.2 % of moisture, 0.5% of protein, 0.1% of fat, 14.1% of carbohydrates, 0.7% of mineral matter, 3.4% of fiber, 0.05% of calcium, 0.02% of potassium, 1.2 mg/100g of iron, 0.2 mg/g of nicotinic acid, phyllemblin, phyllemblic acid, gallic acid, emblicol, quercetin, hydroxymethyl furfural, ellagic acid, pectin, putranjivan *A. emblicannin A* and *B, punigluconin*, penduncul agin (Moeenuddin *et al.*, 2023) and tannins. It has antioxidant, immunomodulatory, antipyretic, analgesic, cytoprotective, antitussive and gastroprotective properties.

Supplementation of amla through water or feed to broilers had shown many positive effects, like improved FCR and body weight gain (Islam *et al.*, 2020), decreased mortality and improved immunity (Abo *et al.*, 2023), decreased abdominal fat percentage, decreased serum total cholesterol level (Begum *et al.*, 2019) decreased gut *E. coli* and S*almonella* count (Islam *et al.*, 2020).

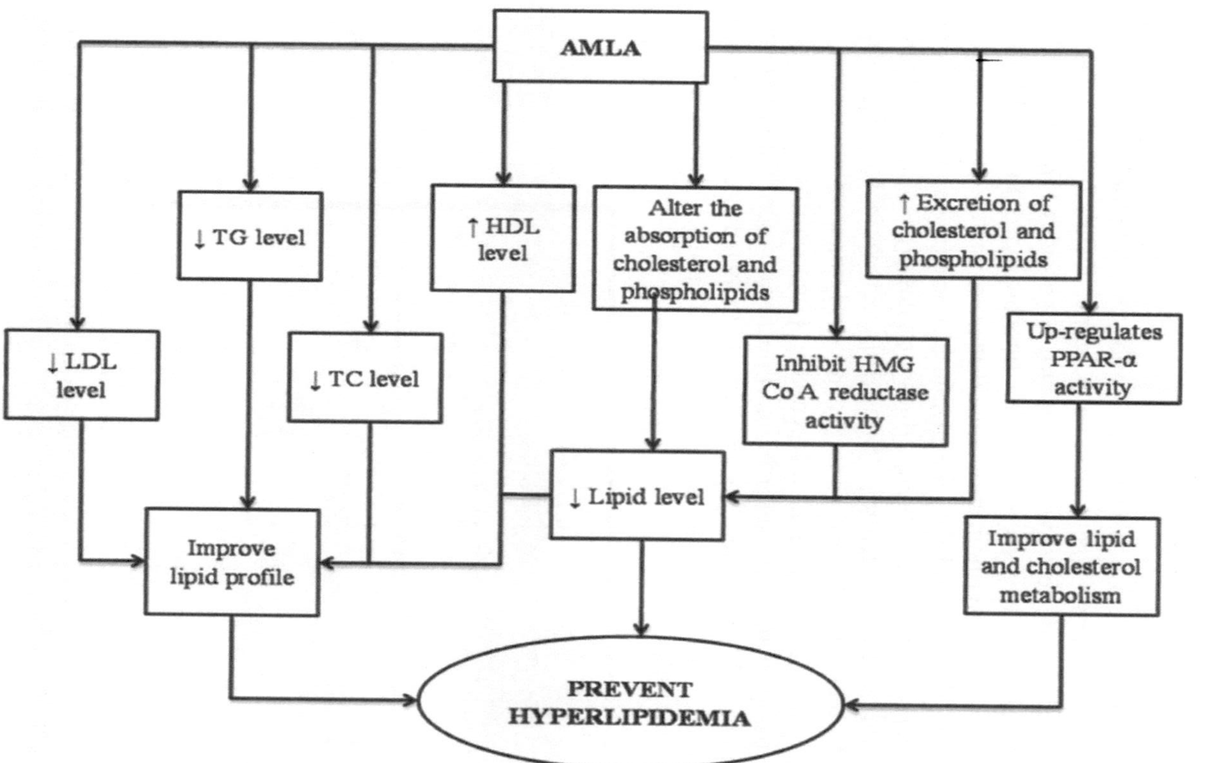

Mechanism of Amla as anti-hyperlipidemic agent (Kaur *et al.*, 2013) (TG-Triglycerides, TC-Total cholesterol, LDL-Low density lipids and HDL-High density lipids)

Giloy

Giloy (*Tinospora cordifolia*) is also known as Guduchi and Amritavalli in Sanskrit, Tippa teega in Telugu, Shindilakodi in Tamil, Amruthaballi in Kannada, Chittamrutu in Malayalam, Gulvel in Marathi, Giloy in Hindi, Garo in Gujarati belongs to Menispermaceae family is a well-known medicinal plant known as panacea (remedy) for all the diseases and disorders in Indian ayurveda (Prajwala *et al.*, 2019).

The major phytochemical constituents in giloy are Alkaloids (Tinosporin, tinosporic acid, berberine, palmitine, tembatarine, mangoflorine , choline, tinosporin, isocolumbin, tetrahydropalmatine), Glycosides (18 Nonderodane glycoside, furanoid diterpene glycoside, tinocordiside, tinocordifoliside, cordioside, syringin, syringinapiosylglycoside, palmatosides C and P, cordifoliside A, B, C, D and E), Diterpenoid lactones (tinosporon columbin, clerodane derivatives, tinosporon, tinosporisides, jateorine, columbin, tinosporal, tinosporide), Steroids (Sitosterol, octacosanol, heptacosanol, nonacosan-15-one, tetrahydrofuran, hydroxyecdysone, makisterone A, giloinsterol, ecdysterone), Sesquiterpenoids (einocordifolin) and some miscellaneous compounds like jatrorrhizine, tinosporidin, cordifol, cordifelone, giloin, giloinin, arabinogalactan (Saeed *et al.*, 2020), heptacosanol, nonacosan, tetrahydrofuran, gilonin, giloinsteroljateorine, clerodane furano diterpene (Joshi and Kaur, 2016).

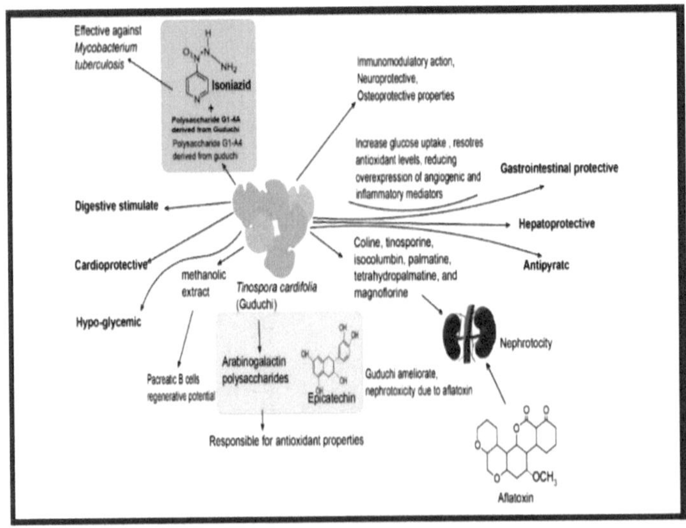

Schematic figure depicting various pharmacological effects of *Tinospora cordifolia* extract (Mishra *et al.*, 2016)

Giloy inclusion to the broiler feed has contributed to improved gain in body weights (Joshi *et al.*, 2015), FCR (Singh *et al.*, 2018), livability (Sachan *et al.*, 2019) and immunity (Bhardwaj *et al.*, 2012).

Improving Digestion and Absorption

Feeding turmeric to broilers increased the digestion and absorption. It's due to the fact that enhanced secretions of amylase, trypsin, chymotrypsin and lipase enzymes (Platel and Srinivasan, 2000) by curcumin present in turmeric. Curcumin also possesses the property of modulating intestinal barrier function (Jabczyk *et al.*, 2021) thus, aids in digestive process and thereby increasing digestion and absorption. Giloy contains different kinds of phytochemicals like tinosporine, β-Amyrin which have hepatoprotective activity (Jain, 2021) and amla contains flavonoids, soluble tannins and gallic acid known to stimulate the digestion system in poultry and improved the function of liver and increased the pancreatic digestive enzymes (Jain, 2021). Presence of above mentioned and other phytochemicals in turmeric, amla and giloy increases digestion and absorption in the broilers hence the feed conversion ratio.

Inhibiting Growth of Pathogenic Bacteria

Curcumin is also known for its antibacterial (Javale and Sabnis, 2010) and prebiotic property which could modulate gut microbiota (Jabczyk *et al.* 2021). Supplementing turmeric to broilers resulted in improved performance associated with significantly increased absorptive capacity of chicken gastrointestinal tract (GIT) due to increased length of small intestine. The prebiotic effect of curcumin inhibits the growth of *Escherichia coli* and *Salmonella*, selectively stimulate the growth of *Lactobacillus* development in the gut. Antibacterial effects of amla on gram negative bacteria and beneficial effect on gram positive bacteria mainly be attributed to alkaloids, cardiac glucosides, saponins, tannins terpenoids, phenols and flavonoids (Javale and Sabnis 2010) resulted in production of more lactic acid by *Lactobacilli* in gut which further led to decreased pH in intestine thereby at low pH *Coliforms* were not able to colonize themselves within intestinal mucosa (Dalal *et al.*, 2018). Giloy consists of arabinogalactan, which serves as a prebiotic helps in promoting beneficial gut habitant bacteria assisting in their repopulation (Li *et al.*, 2015).

Increasing Immune system of Host

Turmeric has the ability to modulate the activation of T cells, B cells, macrophages, neutrophils, natural killer cells, and dendritic cells (Ganesh and Bharat, 2007). Amla also potentiates T cells and macrophages (Marzo *et al.*,

1990) and giloy (*Tinospora cordifolia*) as immune modulator affects IL-1, which stimulates B-cell proliferation and immunoglobulin secretion (Saeed *et al.*, 2020).

By Increasing Intestinal Villus Height and Crypt Depth

Turmeric, amla and giloy supplementation with its antimicrobial and prebiotic properties known to reduce the growth of many pathogenic and non-pathogenic intestinal bacteria which hinder the digestion. The colonization of unwanted bacteria is reduced and beneficial bacteria is improved, hence the gut health. Mustafa *et al.* (2021), Ahsan *et al.* (2022) and several others researchers had observed significant increase in villus height and villus height to crypt depth ratio in small intestine of broilers supplemented with turmeric. Research on supplementing amla and giloy to the broilers regarding intestinal morphology are limited but both of them are known to stimulate and increase the digestion and absorption of feed which might be attributed to increase in villus height and crypt depth in various segments of small intestine of broilers. More the villus height and depth of the intestine more the surface area for absorption.

Conclusion

Owing to the numerous benefits of Turmeric, Amla and Giloy they can be safely included in the broiler diet instead of antibiotic growth promoter. As their inclusion known to improve digestion, absorption, FCR, immune status and gut health of the broilers.

6

Acidifiers
Feed Additives In Broilers

M.G. Nikam[1], K.K. Khose[2], G.R. Gangane[3], A.M. Chappalwar[4] V.K. Munde[5] and Vaishnavi Chormule

[1&2]*Department of Poultry Science*
[3]*Department of Veterinary Pathology*
[4&5]*Department of Livestock Products and Technology*
College of Veterinary and Animal Sciences, Parbhani- 431 402, Maharashtra

The acidifiers could be used to favourably manipulate the intestinal microbial populations and improve the immune response, hence perform an activity similar to antibiotics in feed. Acidifiers also improve the digestibility of nutrients and increases the absorption of minerals. The incorporation of organic acids also leads to thinning of the intestinal lining which facilitates better absorption of nutrients and its efficient utilization. However, their effect will not be similar among all types of organic acids as their mechanism of activity is based on its pKa value. At present, coated salts of acidifiers are available commercially for use in feed of poultry. The role of different acidifiers in poultry nutrition with their potent applications in improving nutrient digestibility, mineral utilization, meat quality, enhancing immunity, antimicrobial effects in countering pathogenic bacteria, boosting performance and production, and thus safeguarding health of poultry.

The acidic specificities of acidifiers as feed additives are attributed to the carboxyl functional group, -COOH of the organic acids, including the fatty and amino acids. They include either simple mono-carboxylic acids (formic, acetic, propionic and butyric acids) or carboxylic acids with the hydroxyl group (lactic, malic, tartaric and citric acids) or short-chain carboxylic acids containing double bonds (fumaric and sorbic acids) (Shahidi *et al.* 2014). The short-chain organic acids (C_1–C_7) have specific antimicrobial activity; however, their effect in pH reduction and antimicrobial activity varies with their dissociation status depending on the specific pKa of each acid. Hence, lower the pKa value, stronger the acid which describe its ability to lower the pH of environment. Most acids used as feed additives have their pKa value between 3 and 5. Many acids are also used as salts of sodium, potassium or calcium, the benefits being less odour, easy handling during feed manufacture, less corrosive and more soluble in water than the free acids (Huyghebaert *et al.* 2011). The inorganic acidifiers under use, particularly hydrochloric, sulphuric and phosphoric acids are cheaper than organic acids but in pure form they are very corrosive and hazardous liquids (Kim *et al.* 2005).

Acidifiers in feed inhibit the growth of pathogenic bacteria and curtail the microbial competition for host nutrients by influencing the pH. The proliferation of most pH sensitive bacteria (*E. coli, Salmonella* and *Clostridium perfringens*) is minimized below pH 5 while acid-tolerant ones survive.

Growth Performance

Daskiran *et al.* (2004) observed that improved broiler performance with supplementation of commercial phosphoric and citric acid based dietary acidifier (Lucta'cid). Dixit (2006) observed significant ($P<0.05$) effect of feed and water acidifiers on growth performance and better economic profit in broiler production. Paul *et al.* (2007) reported that organic acid salts significantly improved ($P<0.05$) feed conversion ratio (FCR) compared with the antibiotic treatment. Singh (2008) observed significant ($P<0.05$) differences on BWG, feed intake and FCR with supplementation of feed acidifier. Adil *et al.* (2010) observed broiler chicken fed diets supplemented with organic acids had significantly ($P<0.05$) improved body weight gains and feed conversion ratio. Ogunwole *et al.* (2011) reported that significantly improved ($P<0.05$) performance of broiler with supplementation of Biotronics SE (an acidifier). Dizaji *et al.* (2012) observed improved ($P<0.05$) in body weight, daily weight gain and better feed conversion ratio with dietary supplementations of prebiotic, probiotic, synbiotic and acidifier in broiler. Brzoska *et al.* (2013) reportedorganic acid acidifier used in this experiment at the rates of 3 to 9 g/kg diet has a growth enhancing and mortality reducing effect in broiler chickens. Fallah and Rezaei (2013) reported that addition of fermacto prebiotic and Biotronic S.E (an acidifier) significantly ($P<0.05$) increased the final body weight of broilers. Hedayati *et al.* (2013) observed that weekly body weight, feed intake and FCR, there was a significant ($P<0.05$) improvement with dietary supplementation of an acidifier in broilers. Marin-Flamand *et al.* (2013) observed an improvement ($P<0.05$) on feed consumption (FC), feed conversion ratio (FCR), and survival rate (SR) as compared to the control with supplementation of organic acid blends (OAB) of ascorbic (A), citric

(C), malic (M), sorbic (S), and tartaric (T) acids through the drinking water in broiler chickens. Kamal and Ragaa (2014) reported non-significant effect on cumulative feed consumption when dietary supplementation of organic acids in broiler chicken.Srinivas *et al.* (2014) observed acidifier alone had shown significantly (P<0.05) higher body weight (2059 g) gain followed by probiotic + MOS combination (2039 g) during the overall experimental period (0-42 d) compared to control and antibiotic broiler chickens. Ali (2015) observed improvement (P<0.05) of the general performance of broiler chicks and lowered mortality rate with supplantation of Biotronics powder (organic acid combination) broiler chicks. Hedayati *et al.* (2015) reported that dietary supplementation of acidifiers (containing citric acid, acetic acid, propionic acid, lactic acid) @0.1% improved (P<0.05) the growth performance in broilers. Ishfaq *et al.* (2015) observed significant (P<0.05) increase in body weight gain and feed conversion ratio was improved with supplementation of Acipure (acidifier) compared with the group of birds fed untreated diets and mortality rate is also lower in treated group. Sohail *et al.* (2015) observed that addition of organic acids (benzoic, acetic and formic) is helpful to significantly (P<0.05) improve weight gain, feed intake and feed conversion ratio of the broiler birds. Al-Sultan *et al.* (2016) observed body weight, weight gain and feed conversion of broiler birds showed significant (P<0.01) improvement with dietary pre, pro, synbiotic and organic acid salt supplementation from 0 to 21D, 22-42 D and from 0-41 D in comparison with the control group. Dousa *et al.* (2016) reported that inclusion of probiotic and probiotic plus acidifier to broiler chicken's diets improved (P<0.05)live body weight. Palamidi *et al.* (2016) reported that acidifiers supplementation in feed improved (P<0.05) the growth performance in broilers. Ahmed *et al.* (2018) reported that body weight, feed consumption and feed conversion ratio were significantly affected (P<0.01) by organic acids and their combination. Roofchaei *et al.* (2019) observed that feed conversion ratio (FCR) was improved (P<0.05) in broiler chickens with supplementation of XG(xylanase and b-glucanase) + acidifier during the entire production period (1 to 35 d) of the trial. Khalil *et al.* (2020) reported that acidifier, lysozyme and combined groups had significantly (P<0.05) higher live body weight and lower feed conversion ratio compared to the control group in broiler.Emili*et al.* (2021) observed that combination of organic acids and essential oil had shown enhanced broiler performance (P<0.05) with better economic returns. Gao *et al.* (2021) reported that diet supplementation with acidifiers could improve (P<0.05) the growth performance in broilers.

Immune Response

Hassan *et al.* (2012) observed that that antibody titer against Newcastle disease virus (NDV) vaccine was increased (P<0.05) with supplementation of Nutrilac (acidifier) in diets of broiler chicken. Hedayati *et al.* (2014) reported that there were non-significant differences among the dietary supplementation of acidifier against antibody titers against Newcastle Disease (ND). Sohail *et al.* (2015) observed that the maximum ND titer value in dietary treated with acidifier groups of broilers. Al-Sultan *et al.* (2016) reported that synbiotic, probiotics, prebiotics and organic acids (acidifier) increases the post vaccination log10 values of NDV antibodies significantly (P<0.01) in serum at 3 weeks post vaccination. Pathak *et al.* (2016) observed antibody titer on Day 35 against Newcastle disease vaccine was higher in acidifier treated group than other groups (P<0.01). Amira *et al.* (2017) observed that increased (P<0.05) immunity against NDV diets supplemented with organic acids in broiler diet.

Carcass Traits

Nourmohammadi *et al.* (2010) observed that numerically decreased relative weight of breast, thighs and back with supplemented of citric acid in broiler diet. Ogunwole *et al.* (2011) reported that non-significant effect on carcass and internal organs weights were the inclusion of AGP or acidifier in the diets of broiler. Abu *et al.* (2013) reported that carcass yield was non-significantly affected with acidifier in a blood meal-based diet on broilers. Brzoska *et al.* (2013) observed non-significant effect on relative weight of breast and leg muscles, gizzard, liver and carcass depot fat percentage by dietary acidifier treatments in broiler. Fallah and Rezaei, (2013) reported that addition of fermacto prebiotic and Biotronic S.E in diet to decreased (P<0.05) abdominal fat and increased carcass weight in broilers. Srinivas *et al.* (2014) observed that dietary supplements did not have significant effect on various carcass parameters, except for abdominal fat percentage, which was significantly (P<0.05) lower in probiotic alone and acidifier + MOS groups, while the rest of the treatment groups did not differ from control. Ali (2015) reported non-significant difference between groups in dressing percentage and non-carcass components (heart, gizzard and liver) in broiler. Sohail *et al.* (2015) observed non-significant effect on dressing percentage, breast meat, thigh meat and giblet organs weight e.g., liver, heart in broilers. Youssef *et al.* (2017) found that the percentage of carcass yield did not show any significant effect due to dietary treatments, but exhibited a numerical improve in probiotic group (72.84%), followed by lactic acid and antibiotic groups (71.45%) in comparison with the normal group (70.35%). Malik *et al.* (2018) reported addition of bacillus subtilis, acidifiers and their combination did not show any significant effect in net carcass, dressing percentage and the relative weight of internal organs. Nikmah *et al.* (2021) observed a mixture of probiotics and acidifier at the level of 0.3% showed a positive effect on decreasing ($P<0.05$) the percentage of abdominal fat from 1.52% to 1.35%.

Economics

Thirumeigmanam *et al.* (2006) observed lower cost of production per kg live weight in broilers on diet supplemented with organic acids than those fed with basal diet and antibiotic supplemented diet. Adil *et al.* (2010) reported that dietary supplementation of organic acids was economically better and an extra profit of Rs. 3.49 per chick was achieved in the group fed diet supplemented with 2 percent fumaric acid followed by Rs. 2.87 in the group fed with 2 percent lactic acid in the diet. Alzawqari *et al.* (2013) reported that addition of citric acid in the drinking water 8 hour before slaughter could reduce intestinal microflora colonization and might be a fruitful strategy against bacterial contamination of broiler products during processing and thus increasing the profit. Menconi *et al.* (2013) revealed that organic acid product might improved animal welfare and economic concerns in the poultry industry by reducing body weight loss and improving meat quality attributes. Sadeghi *et al.* (2014) reported increased returns to investment due to addition of organic acid in broiler diet. Venkatasubramani *et al.* (2014) observed that addition of combination of formic and propionic acids at 0.1 percent level in the diet of broilers was economically beneficial and comparable to the antibiotic fed group and advocated the use of organic acids in the diet of broilers to replace antibiotic growth promoters.

Conclusions

The addition of acidifier in feed should significantly ($P<0.05$) used as an alternative to antibiotics to improved commercial broiler performance, immune response and economics.Through beneficial antimicrobial effect of acidifier to good gut environment and overall health benefits to broiler birds.

References

Abu, O. A., Ogunwole, O. A., Adedeji, B. S., Adeboboye, A. V. K., and Tewe, O. O., 2013. Growth and carcass characteristics of finishing broilers on acidified blood meal-based diet.African Journal of Livestock Extension, 11.

Adil, S., Banday, T., Bhat, G. A., Mir, M. S., and Rehman, M., 2010. Effect of dietary supplementation of organic acids on performance, intestinal histomorphology, and serum biochemistry of broiler chicken. Veterinary Medicine International.

Adil S, Banday MT, Bhat GA, Khan I and Bhatt MI (2010). A study on the profitability of broiler chicken fed diets supplemented with organic acids. Indian Journal of Poultry Science, 45(2): 220-223.

Ahmed, A., M. V. Dhumal., M. G. Nikam., P. V. Nandedkar and V. S. Ingle., 2018. Effect of Supplementation of Organic Acids and Their Combination as an Alternative to Antibiotic Growth Promoter on Performance, Gut Health, Immune Status and Economics of Broiler Production. International Journal of Livestock Research, 9 (02), 154-165.

Al-Sultan, S. I., Abdel-Raheem, S. M., El-Ghareeb, W. R., and Mohamed, M. H., 2016. Comparative effects of using prebiotic, probiotic, synbiotic and acidifier on growth performance, intestinal microbiology and histomorphology of broiler chicks. Japanese Journal of Veterinary Research, 64(2), 187-195.

Ali, A. S. A., 2015. Comparative Study Effect of Biotronic as Natural Acidifier with Antibiotic on Broiler Performance Values. M. Sc Thesis, submitted to Sudan University of Science and Technology.

Alzawqari MH, Kermanshahi H, Moghaddam H N, Tawassoli MH and Gilani A (2013). Alteration of gut microflora through citric acid treated drinking water in preslaughter male broilers. African Journal of Microbiology Research, 7(7): 564-567.

Amira, A. E. H., Kamel, E. R., Abo-Salem, M. E., and Atallah, S. T., 2017. Comparative Study on the Effect of Organic Acids, Prebiotics and Enzymes Supplementation on Broiler Chicks Economic and Productive Efficiency. Benha Journal of Applied Sciences, 2(1), 1-8.

Brzoska, F., Sliwinski, B., and Michalik-Rutkowska, O., 2013. Effect of dietary acidifier on growth, mortality, post-slaughter parameters and meat composition of broiler chickens. Ann. Animal Science, 13(1), 85-96.

Daskiran, M., Teeter, R. G., Vanhooser, S. L., Gibson, M. L., and Roura, E., 2004. Effect of dietary acidification on mortality rates, general performance, carcass characteristics, and serum chemistry of broilers exposed to cycling high ambient temperature stress. Journal of Applied Poultry Research, 13(4), 605-613.

Dixit, V.A., 2006. Comparative studies on effect of water and feed acidifiers on performance of broilers. M.V.Sc. Thesis, submitted to Maharashtra Animal and Fishery Sciences University, Nagpur.

Dizaji, B. R., Hejazi, S., and Zakeri, A., 2012. Effects of dietary supplementations of prebiotics, probiotics, synbiotics and acidifiers on growth performance and organs weights of broiler chicken. European Journal of Experimental Biology, 2(6), 2125-2129.

Dousa, B. M., Adam, M. S., Malik, H. E., Ali, O. H., Elamin, K. M., and Elagib, H. A., 2016. Impact of probiotics and acidifiers on growth performance and blood chemistry of broiler chickens.

Emili, V. R., Balakrishnan, U., Yasir, B., and Chandrasekar, S., 2021. Effect of dietary supplementation of acidifiers and essential oils on growth performance and intestinal health of broiler. Journal of Applied Poultry Research, 30(3), 100179.

Fallah, R., and Rezaei, H., 2013. Effect of dietary prebiotic and acidifier supplementation on the growth performance, carcass characteristics and serum biochemical parameters of broilers. Journal of Cell and Animal Biology, 7(3), 21-24.

Gao, C. Q., Shi, H. Q., Xie, W. Y., Zhao, L. H., Zhang, J. Y., Ji, C., and Ma, Q. G., 2021. Dietary supplementation with acidifiers improves the growth performance, meat quality and intestinal health of broiler chickens. Animal Nutrition.

Hassan, E. R., Zeinab, K. M. K. M. E., Girh, M. A., and Mekky, H. M., 2012. Comparative studies between the effects of antibiotic (oxytetracycline); probiotic and acidifier on E. coli infection and immune response in broiler chickens. Journal of American Science, 8(4), 795-801.

Hedayati, M., Manafi, M., Khalaji, S., Yari, M., Esapour, A., Nazari, E., and Mohebi, F., 2015. Combination effect of probiotic and organic acids on blood biochemistry and immunity parameters of broilers. International Journal of Agriculture Innovations and Research, 3(4), 1288-1293.

Hedayati, M., Manafi, M., Yari, M., and Avara, A., 2014. The influence of an Acidifier feed additive on biochemical parameters and immune response of broilers. Annual Research & Review in Biology, 4(10)1637-1645.

Hedayati, M., Manafi, M., Yari, M., and Vafaei, P., 2013. Effects of supplementing diets with an acidifier on performance parameters and visceral organ weights of broilers. European Journal of Zoological Research, 2(6), 49-55.

Huyghebaert, G., Ducatelle, R., and Van Immerseel, F., 2011. An update on alternatives to antimicrobial growth promoters for broilers. The Veterinary Journal, 187(2), 182-188.

Ishfaq, A., Rather, S. A., Mir, A. H., and Gupta, M., 2015. Effect of Acipure (feed acidifier) on the growth performance, mortality and gut pH of broiler chickens. IJLR, 5(10), 40-46.

Kamal, A. M., and Ragaa, N. M., 2014. Effect of dietary supplementation of organic acids on performance and serum biochemistry of broiler chicken. Nature and Science, 12(2), 38-45.

Khalil, K. K. I., Islam, M. A., Sujan, K. M., Mustari, A., Ahamd, N., and Miah, M. A., 2020. Dietary acidifier and lysozyme improve growth performances and hemato-biochemical profile in broiler chicken. Journal of Advanced Biotechnology and Experimental Therapeutics, 3(3), 241-247.

Kim, Y. Y., Kil, D. Y., Oh, H. K., and Han, I. K., 2005. Acidifier as an alternative material to antibiotics in animal feed. Asian-Australasian journal of animal sciences, 18(7), 1048-1060.

Malik, H. E., Hafzalla, R. H., H A, A. O., M O, E. M., Dousa, B. M., Ali, A. M., and Elamin, K. M., 2018. Effect of probiotics and acidifiers on carcass yield, internal organs, cuts and meat to bone ratio of broiler chicken. IOSR Journal of Agriculture and Veterinary Science, 9(12), 18-23.

Marin-Flamand, E., Vázquez-Durán, A., and Méndez-Albores, A., 2013. Effect of organic acid blends in drinking water on growth performance, blood constituents and immune response of broiler chickens. The Journal of Poultry Science, 51(2), 144-150.

Menconi A, Kuttappan VA, Hernandez-Velasco X, Urbano T , Matté F, Layton S, Kallapura G, Latorre J, Morales B E, Prado O, Vicente JL, Barton J, Andreatti Filho RL, Lovato M, Hargis BM and Tellez G (2013). Evaluation of a commercially available organic acid product on body weight loss, carcass yield, and meat quality during preslaughter feed withdrawal in broiler chickens: A poultry welfare and economic perspective. Journal of Poultry Science, 2(93): 448-455.

Nikmah, A., Ridhana, F., Fitri, I., and Hikmah, H., 2021. Effects of Fermentated Feed and Probiotic + Acidifier Supplements on Glucose Levels and Abdomen Chicken Fat Broiler. Budapest International Research in Exact Sciences (BirEx) Journal, 3(2), 126-134.

Nourmohammadi, R., Hosseini, S. M., and Farhangfar, H., 2010. Influence of citric acid and microbial phytase on growth performance and carcass characteristics of broiler chickens. American Journal of Animal and Veterinary Sciences, 5(4), 282-288.

Ogunwole, O. A., Abu, O. A., and Adepoju, I. A., 2011. Performance and carcass characteristics of broiler finishers fed acidifier-based diets. Pak J Nut, 10, 631-636.

Palamidi, I., Paraskeuas, V., Theodorou, G., Breitsma, R., Schatzmayr, G., Theodoropoulos, G., and Mountzouris, K. C., 2016. Effects of dietary acidifier supplementation on broiler growth performance, digestive and immune function indices. Animal Production Science, 57(2), 271-281.

Pathak, M., Mandal, G. P., Patra, A. K., Samanta, I., Pradhan, S., and Haldar, S., 2016. Effects of dietary supplementation of cinnamaldehyde and formic acid on growth performance, intestinal microbiota and immune response in broiler chickens. Animal Production Science, 57(5), 821-827.

Paul, S. K., Samanta, G., Halder, G., and Biswas, P., 2007. Effect of a combination of organic acid salts as antibiotic replacer on the performance and gut health of broiler chickens. Livestock Research for Rural Development, 19(11), 2007.

Roofchaei, A., Rezaeipour, V., Vatandour, S., and Zaefarian, F., 2019. Influence of dietary carbohydrases, individually or in combination with phytase or an acidifier, on performance, gut morphology and microbial population in broiler chickens fed a wheat-based diet. Animal Nutrition, 5(1), 63-67.

Sadeghi GH, Janfadah M and Moslehi S (2014). Effects of a commercial mixture of herbal essential oils and vitamins (Provital Reg.) and an organic acid (Totacid Reg.) on performance and economical efficiency in broilers. Journal of Medicinal Plants Research, 8(12): 475-478.

Shahidi, S., Maziar, Y., and Delaram, N. Z. 2014. Influence of dietary organic acids supplementation on reproductive performance of freshwater Angelfish (Pterophyllum scalare). Journal of Global Veterinarian, 13(3), 373–377.

Singh, A. K., and Nagar, A., 2020. Effect of cardamom and ginger powder supplementation on body weight gain and feed efficiency in caged broilers. International Journal of Current Microbiology and Applied Sciences, 9(8), 2159-2168.

Singh, V.K., 2008. Studies on the efficacy of the different feed acidifier on performance of broiler birds challenged with E.coli infection. M.V.Sc. Thesis, submitted to Maharashtra Animal and Fishery Sciences University, Nagpur.

Sohail, R., Saeed, M., Chao, S., Soomro, R. N., Arain, M. A., Abbasi, I. H. R., and Yousaf, M., 2015. Comparative effect of different organic acids (benzoic, acetic and formic) on growth performance, immune response and carcass traits of broilers. J Anim Prod Adv, 5, 757-764.

Srinivas, G., Preetam, V. C., Qudratullah, S., Raju, M. V. L. N., and Reddy, M. R., 2014. The effect of dietary supplementation of probiotic, prebiotic and acidifier in comparison to antibiotic on performance and carcass traits of broilers. Indian Journal of Poultry Science, 49(1), 7-10.

Thirumeigmanam D, Swain RK, Mohanty SP and Pati PK (2006). Effect of dietary supplementation of organic acids on performance of broiler chicken. Indian Journal of Animal Nutrition, 23(1): 34-40.

Venkatasubramani R, Vasanthakumar P, Chandrasekaran D, Rajendran D and Purushothaman MR (2014). Performance of broilers fed formic and propionic acid supplemented diets. Animal Nutrition and Feed Technology, 14(1): 81-90.

7

β-glucans
An Alternative to Antibiotics in Broiler

M.G. Nikam[1], K.K. Khose[1], G.R. Gangane[2], A.M. Chappalwar[3] V.K. Munde[4] and Vaishnavi Chormule

[1]Department of Poultry Science
[2]Department of Veterinary Pathology
[3]Department of Livestock Products Technology
[4]Department of Animal Nutrition
College of Veterinary and Animal Sciences, Parbhani- 431402, Maharashtra

---

β-glucans are carbohydrates made of complex glucose polymers that provides the major structure found in the cell wall of yeast, fungi, algae, and cereal grains such as oats and barley. The structures of β-glucans vary depending on the original source and the type of linkages present on the glucose polymers. β-glucans consist of a backbone of glucose molecules linked at the 1 and 3 carbon atoms (Jacob and Pescatore, 2017). The six-sided glucose rings are connected together in linear or branched forms with glycosidic linkages. The structure of these glycosidic linkages will affect the functionality of the β-glucan molecules. The β-glucans may play a role in replacing antibiotics and stimulating the immune system. It was reported that β-glucan was effective in promoting growth of broiler chickens and improving meat quality.

The use of β-glucans is generally more widely accepted by consumers than antibiotics even at low dose. β-glucans from the yeast cell wall and mushrooms have been shown to stimulate both specific and non-specific immune responses and improve the chicken growth performance and quality of meat. β-glucans derived from yeast and fungi, so-called β-(1→3) and (1→6)-β-glucans, have been shown to exert beneficial effects when administered as feed supplement to poultry.

Table 1: Types of β-glucan linkages generally found in different sources

Source	Linkage
Bacteria	(1→3)
Fungal	(1→3) (1→6) with short branches
Yeast	(1→3) (1→6) with longer branches
Cereal (barley and oats)	(1→3) (1→4)

Results of the Recent Experiments on use of β-glucans in Broiler Diets

Cheng *et al.* (2004) reported that non-significant differences in weight gain and feed efficiency with β-glucans supplementation at 0, 0.012, 0.025 or 0.05% in broiler diets. Chae *et al.* (2006) observed non-significant effect of β-glucans at 0%, 0.02% and 0.04% on growth performance in broilers. Rathgeber *et al.* (2008) reported that yeast β-glucans were as effective in promoting growth of broiler chickens as virginiamycin, an antibiotic routinely added to broiler diets at sub therapeutic levels. Shendare *et al.* (2008) concluded that the effect of the inclusion of Manno-Oligosaccharide & β-glucans (AGRIMOS) @ 1Kg / ton of feed in broiler shows significantly (P<0.01) higher body weight gain & improvement in feed efficiency as compared to the control diet. Zhang *et al.* (2008) reported that dietary β-1,3/1,6-glucan supplementation at 0, 25, 50, 75, 100 and 125 mg/kg in feed had significantly improved (P<0.05) in body weight gain, feed consumption and feed conversation rate on 21 and 42 days in broiler birds.Lopez *et al.* (2009) was observed that no significant differences in addition of yeast cell wall (YCW); β-1, 3/1, 6-glucan (BG); and mannoprotein complex (MP) purified fractions on broiler performance. Cox *et al.* (2010) reported that non-significant effect of yeast derived β-glucans (Auxoferm YGT) on broiler body weight, body weight gain, feed intake and feed conversion ratio. Rajapakse *et al.* (2010) who reported that the mean body weight of the β-glucans treated group was significantly (P<0.05) higher than that of the control group. Awaad *et al.* (2011) reported that combination of β-glucans and MOS at higher dose level (i.e 2kg/ton) has expressed non-significant differences (P<0.05) on body weights compared with control after 5 week of age. Keser *et al.* (2011) observed that no significant differences in supplementation of β-glucans @ 0.05-0.1% addition into diets containing organic zinc on body weight, average daily gain, feed intake and FCR of broilers during 42 days. Cho *et al.* (2013) reported that inclusion of 0.1% β-glucans would improve (P<0.05) growth performance in broiler chickens. Cheraghi *et al.* (2014) observed that significantly increased (P<0.05) in weight gain, feed intake and feed conversion ratio with broiler birds supplemented with yeast extracted β-glucans and α-mannans (Alphamune) at 0.5, 0.75, 1 or 1.25 g/kg in feed. Moon *et al.* (2016) concluded that use of β-glucan @ 60 ppm can be a potential alternative to antibiotics to improve (P<0.05) the survival rate and performance of broilers. Tian *et al.* (2016) reported that significantly (P<0.05) improved body weight and feed conversion ratio with diet supplemented yeast β-glucans at different levels in broiler chickens. Tawab *et al.* (2019) observed supplementation with 0.015% β-glucans to the diets had negative effects on performance parameters of Ross broilers. Fadl *et al.* (2020) reported that significantly (P<0.05) increased the body weight and total gain weight with dietary supplementation of Mannan-oligosaccharide (MOS) and β-Glucan (Agrimos) on broilers challenged with *Escherichia coli*. Fan *et al.* (2020) observed that the body weight, average daily gain, feed intake and FCR was not affected by the treatments of β-glucans @ 100mg/kg of diet in broilers. Taye *et al.* (2021) reported that β-glucans @5g/100kg and Mos @50g/100kg of feed alone or in combination trough feed was beneficial (P<0.01) by considering overall performance in broilers.

Results of the Recent Experiments with use of β-glucans on Immune Response of Broilers

Guo *et al.* 2003 observed Dietary supplementation with β-glucans from the yeast *Saccharomyces cerevisiae* has been shown to increase phagocytic activity in broiler chicks. Cheng *et al.*(2004) observed that non-significant difference in antibody titer with supplementation of β-glucans at 0, 0.012, 0.025 or 0.05%. An *et al.* (2008) reported that antibody titers against Newcastle disease or infectious bronchitis virus in the chicks fed diets containing β-glucan at 0.025, 0.05 or 0.1% were significantly higher (P<0.05) than in the control. Chen *et al.* 2008 reported that supplementation with yeast β-glucans enhanced the chick's Défense against SE by directly up regulating both the phagocytosis and bactericidal activity of abdominal macrophages. Zhang *et al.* (2008) observed that an enhanced (P<0.05) immunological response at supplemented level of 50 mg/kg of β-1,3/1,6-glucan. Lopez *et al.* (2009) reported that antibody response of Newcastle disease virus vaccine was not affected by dietary addition of yeast cell wall (YCW) β-1, 3/1, 6-glucan (BG). Sadeghi *et al.* (2013) reported that dietary inclusion of prebiotic-based mannan-oligosaccharide and β-glucans has non-significant effect on means of antibody titers against Newcastle and infectious bursal viruses at 21 and 42 days of age. Mahdi (2014) observed that antibody titer to NDV showed that there significant (P< 0.05) differences among all groups at 7, 14 and 21 days of age with supplanted of β-glucans 225μg/ml in drinking water to broiler chicken. Tawab *et al.* (2019) reported that significant effect of β-glucans on innate and adaptive immune responses of broilers vaccinated for routine vaccination with

Newcastle disease virus (NDV) and Avian Influenza H9N2 (AIV) vaccines. Fadl *et al.* (2020) observed significant difference (P<0.05) in HI titer against Newcastle disease (ND) with the supplementation of Mannan-oligosaccharide and β-glucan (Agrimos) through feed in broiler birds. Muthusamy *et al.* (2020) reported haemagglutination inhibition (HI) titer was significantly increased (P<0.05) in diets supplemented with β-glucans in boilers.

Conclusions

β-glucans supplementation in broiler feed was shown to significantly increase (P<0.05) the growth performance and also been shown to enhance immune response by altering the cytokine profiles of broilers. β-Glucans, therefore, may provide a tool for producers trying to reduce or eliminate the use of antibiotics in poultry diets.

References

An, B. K., Cho, B. L., You, S. J., Paik, H. D., Chang, H. I., Kim, S. W., and Kang, C. W. 2008. Growth performance and antibody response of broiler chicks fed yeast derived β-glucan and single-strain probiotics. Asian-Australasian Journal of Animal Sciences, 21(7), 1027-1032.

Awaad, M. H. H., Atta, A. M., El-Ghany, W. A., Elmenawey, M., Ahmed, K., Hassan, A. A., and Kawkab, A. A., 2011. Effect of a specific combination of mannan-oligosaccharides and β-glucans extracted from yeast cell wall on the health status and growth performance of ochratoxicated broiler chickens. Journal of American Science, 7(3), 82-96.

Chae, B. J., Lohakare, J. D., Moon, W. K., Lee, S. L., Park, Y. H., and Hahn, T. W., 2006. Effects of supplementation of β-glucans on the growth performance and immunity in broilers. Research in Veterinary Science, 80(3), 291-298.

Chen, K.L., B.C. Weng, M.T. Chang, Y.H. Liao and T.T. Chen, (2008). Direct enhancement of the phagocytic and bactericidal capability of abdominal macrophage of chicks by β-1,3-1,6-glucans. Poult. Sci., 87: 2242-2249.

Cheng, Y. H., Lee, D. N., Wen, C. M., and Weng, C. F., (2004). Effects of β-glucan supplementation on lymphocyte proliferation, macrophage chemo taxis and specific immune responses in broilers. Asian-Australasian Journal of Animal Sciences, 17(8), 1145-1149.

Cheraghi, A., Khosravinia, H., Mousavi, S. M., and Massori, B., 2014. Effects of dietary levels of yeast extracted β-glucans and α-mannans (Alphamune TM) on performance of broiler chicken raised in normal and thermal-stressed conditions. Poult. Sci, 78, 63-68.

Cho, J. H., Zhang, Z. F., and Kim, I. H., 2013. Effects of single or combined dietary supplementation of β-glucans and kefir on growth performance, blood characteristics and meat quality in broilers. British Poultry Science, 54(2), 216-221.

Cox, C. M., Sumners, L. H., Kim, S., McElroy, A. P., Bedford, M. R., and Dalloul, R. A., 2010. Immune responses to dietary β-glucans in broiler chicks during an Eimeria challenge. Journal of Poultry Science, 89(12), 2597-2607.

Fadl, S. E., El-Gammal, G. A., Sakr, O. A., Salah, A. A., Atia, A. A., Prince, A. M., and Hegazy, A. M., (2020). Impact of dietary Mannan-oligosaccharide and β-glucans supplementation on growth, histopathology, E-coli colonization and hepatic transcripts of TNF-α and NF-κB of broiler challenged with E. coli O_{78}. BMC Veterinary Research, 16(1), 1-14.

Fallah, R., and Rezaei, H., 2013. Effect of dietary prebiotic and acidifier supplementation on the growth performance, carcass characteristics and serum biochemical parameters of broilers. Journal of Cell and Animal Biology, 7(3), 21-24.

Fan, Q., Abouelezz, K. F. M., Wang, Y., Lin, X., Li, L., Gou, Z., and Jiang, S., 2020. Influence of vitamin E, tryptophan and β-glucans on growth performance, meat quality, intestinal immunity, and anti oxidative status of yellow-feathered chickens fed thermally oxidized oils. Livestock Science, 241, 104188.

Guo, Y., R.A. Ali and M.A. Qureshi, (2003). The influence of β-glucan on immune responses in broiler chicks. Immunopharmacol Immunotoxicol, 25(3): 461-472.

Jacob, J., and Pescatore, A. J., 2017. Glucans and the poultry immune system. American Journal of Immunology, 13(1), 45.

Keser, O., Bilal, T., Kutay, H. C., Abas, I., and Eseceli, H., (2012). Effects of Chitosan Oligosaccharide and/or beta-glucans supplementation to diets containing organic zinc on performance and some blood indices in broilers. Pakistan Veterinary Journal, 32(1), 15-19.

Lopez, M. R., Auclair, E., Garcia, F., Esteve-Garcia, E., and Brufau, J., (2009). Use of yeast cell walls; β-1, 3/1, 6-glucans; and mannoproteins in broiler chicken diets. Poultry Science, 88(3), 601-607.

Mahdi, N. R., (2014). Effects of soluble β-glucans on the immune responses of broiler chickens vaccinated with Newcastle disease vaccine and reared under heat stress. Iraqi Journal of Veterinary Medicine, 38(1), 30-39.

Moon, S. H., Lee, I., Feng, X., Lee, H. Y., Kim, J., and Ahn, D. U., (2016). Effect of dietary beta-glucans on the performance of broilers and the quality of broiler breast meat. Asian-Australasian Journal of Animal Sciences, 29 (3), 384.

Muthusamy, G., Joardar, S. N., Samanta, I., Isore, D. P., Roy, B., and Maiti, T. K., (2020). Dietary administered purified β-glucans of edible mushroom (Pleurotus florida) provides immuno stimulation and protection in broiler experimentally challenged with virulent Newcastle disease virus. The Journal of Basic and Applied Zoology, 81(1), 1-10.

Rajapakse, J. R., Buddhika, M. D. P., Nagataki, M., Nomura, H., Watanabe, Y., Ikeue, Y., and Agatsuma, T., (2010). Effect of Sophy β-glucans on immunity and growth performance in broiler chicken. Journal of Veterinary Medical Science, 72 (12), 1629-1632.

Rathgeber, B. M., Budgell, K. L., MacIsaac, J. L., Mirza, M. A., and Doncaster, K. L., (2008). Growth performance and spleen and bursa weight of broilers fed yeast beta-glucan. Canadian Journal of Animal Science, 88(3), 469-473.

Sadeghi, A. A., Mohammadi, A., Shawrang, P., and Aminafshar, M., (2013). Immune responses to dietary inclusion of prebiotic-based mannan-oligosaccharide and β-glucans in broiler chicks challenged with Salmonella enteritidis. Turkish Journal of Veterinary and Animal Sciences, 37(2), 206-213.

Shendare, R. C., Gongle, M. A., Rajput, A. B., Wanjari, B. V., and Mandlekar, S. M., (2008). Effect of supplementation of manno-oligosaccharide and b-glucans on maize-based meal on commercial broilers. Veterinary World, 1(1), 13-15.

Singh, A. K., and Nagar, A., (2020). Effect of cardamom and ginger powder supplementation on body weight gain and feed efficiency in caged broilers. International Journal of Current Microbiology and Applied Sciences, 9 (8), 2159-2168.

Tawab, A. E., Awaad, A., Elnaggar, O. M. A. A., and Elsissi, A. F., (2019). The impact of β glucans on the immune response of broiler chickens vaccinated with NDV and AI H9V Vaccines. Benha Veterinary Medical Journal, 36(2), 100-108.

Taye, K., M.G. Nikam., M.V. Dhumal., K.K. Khose., and V.K. Munde., (2021). Influence of β-glucan, mannan-oligosaccharides and their combination on performance of broiler chicken. International Journal of Livestock Research, 11(11) 26-32.

Tian, X., Shao, Y., Wang, Z., and Guo, Y., (2016). Effects of dietary yeast β-glucans supplementation on growth performance, gut morphology, intestinal Clostridium perfringens population and immune response of broiler chickens challenged with necrotic enteritis. Animal Feed Science and Technology, 215, 144-155.

Zhang, B., Guo, Y., and Wang, Z., (2008). The modulating Effect of β-1, 3/1, 6-glucan supplementation in the diet on performance and immunological responses of broiler chickens. Asian-Australasian Journal of Animal Sciences, 21(2), 237-244.

8

Sodium Butyrate A Novel Feed Additive in Poultry

Kadam, M.M.[1], Bhaisare D.B.[1], Pawar, O.K.[1], Aswathi, P.B.[2] Bokade, H.S.[1] and Vaishnavi Chormule

[1]*Department of Poultry Science, Nagpur Veterinary College, Nagpur Maharashtra*

[2]*Department of Poultry Science, College of Veterinary and Animal Sciences Pookode, Wayanad, Kerala*

Antibiotics have been used since their discovery to cure illness at therapeutic levels and to boost animal feed production at subtherapeutic levels by promoting animal development. Antibiotics have been regarded as necessary additives or supplements for improved growth and preservation of a healthy intestinal ecology in the production of chicken for more than 50 years (Huyghebaert *et al.*, 2011). The Indian government outlawed the use of antibiotics in poultry feed in 2019. (Colistin, for example, is no longer allowed in poultry feed.) As a result, a lot of effort is being put into creating antibiotic substitutes. Alternatives to antibiotics should ideally possess the same advantageous qualities. Many studies have been conducted to find alternatives to isolated nutrients (such as amino acids, fatty acids, minerals, and vitamins), dietary supplements (such as probiotics, prebiotics, synbiotics, organic acids, antioxidants, and enzymes), herbal products (such as polyphenols, herbs, and spices), and genetically modified foods (Das *et al.*, 2012). Numerous feed additives and active components, such as pre- and probiotics, essential oils, short- and medium-chain fatty acids and their salts, enzymes, and others, have several beneficial impacts on the environment of the animal's gastrointestinal tract (GIT) (Gadde *et al.*, 2017). Nevertheless, the mode of action is frequently poorly explained, and the outcomes are inconsistent. Furthermore, studies conducted on them are frequently restricted to particular scenarios, which makes it challenging for experts to assess whether the results seen may be repeated in field settings using alternative genetic lines, feed components, formulations, etc.

Among these alternatives, Organic acids are a well-liked substitute that are thought to be appropriate for usage in animal feeds. These substances are characterized as short-chain fatty acids that specifically promote the growth or activity of advantageous bacterial species, hence providing advantages to the host by eliminating detrimental bacterial populations present in the fowl digestive system. These are byproducts of the fermentation of carbohydrates in mammalian intestines or microbial metabolism. The three most well-known organic acids are butyric acid, propionic acid, and acetic acid; these are sometimes referred to as short-chain fatty acids (SCFAs) or volatile fatty acids (VFAs). Butyric acid has one noteworthy characteristic among them. Short-chain fatty acids like butyric acid have a variety of advantageous impacts on animals. In animal nutrition, its derivatives—sodium and calcium salts, as well as mono-, di-, and triglycerides—are frequently utilized. The most well-researched of these is sodium butyrate, which has been shown to change bacterial populations in the intestine and caecum as well as lengthen GIT villi in animals (Chamba *et al.*, 2014; Fernández-Rubio *et al.*, 2009; Bortoluzzi *et al.*, 2017). Its density is 0.958 g/ml, its molecular weight is 88.12 g/mol, and its pKa is 4.82. However, because butyric acid is naturally volatile and caustic, using the sodium salt of butyric acid makes it more stable and easier to handle.

Mode of Action

PHASE 1: Sodium butyrate break down into sodium ion and butyrate and forms butyric acid after ingestion.

PHASE 2: As the crop, proventriculus, and gizzard has an acidic pH, it allows butyric acid to stay in its un-dissociated form. Butyric acid modulates MUC gene expression in goblet cells which improves the properties of the mucus layer thus improves the protection of the gizzard.

PHASE 3: When butyric acid enters the proximal small intestine, it will dissociate into butyrate and hydrogen ions. Here, butyric acid is readily assimilated by enterocytes via passive transport and used to increase villus length and cells turnover.

STAGE 4: However, due to the higher pH in this environment, butyric acid becomes divided into butyrate ions which can be absorbed as a source of energy as well, which require different methods for their absorption.

→ Via diffusion

→ Via HCO3- exchange method

→ Via active transport (MCT1 & SMCT1)

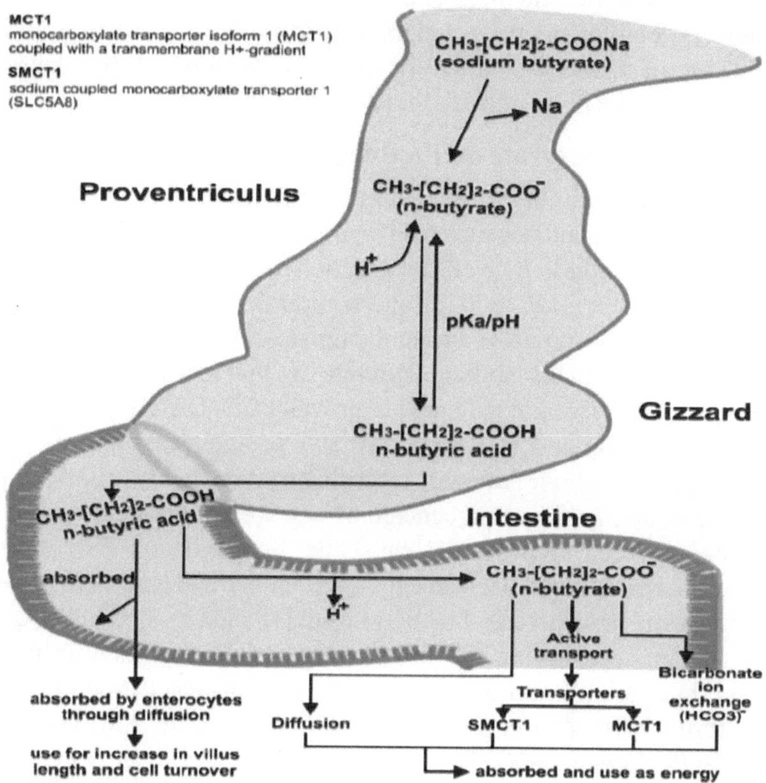

Source: World Poultry Science Journal

However, the enterocytes' preferred energy source is butyric acid. The only solution for the antibacterial effect is this butyric acid, which is robustly lipophilic and capable of diffusing through bacterial membranes. By lowering the stomach pH and speeding up the transformation of pepsinogen into pepsin, adding SB to chicken diets can improve the rate at which nutrients including minerals, proteins, and amino acids are absorbed (Youn *et al.*, 2005). By reducing metabolic energy, decreasing cell membrane metabolism, allowing cellular fluids to escape, and obstructing the use of nutrients, this low pH kills harmful bacteria (Kirchgessner and Roth, 1982). Therefore, reducing the amount of harmful bacteria in the chicken intestine is the primary goal of dietary SB supplementation.

Why Coated Sodium Butyrate

- Uncoated butyric acid has the ability to have bactericidal effects in the proximal gut, limiting the amount of bacteria that travels to the distal intestine and, consequently, the bacterial challenge there.

- Because butyric acid must be undissociated in order to have bactericidal effects, employing protected or coated sodium butyrate permits the release of undissociated butyric acid into the hindgut, but the released butyric acid will quickly dissociate.

Effect of Sodium Butyrate on Productive Performance

Butyrate, also known as butyric acid, has been proven to have positive impacts on broiler production indices such feed intake, weight gain, and feed conversion rate (FCR) in addition to its well-documented health benefits (Antongiovanni *et al.*, 2007; Leeson *et al.*, 2005; Taherpour *et al.*, 2009). In comparison to positive and negative controls during the finisher phase, Chamba *et al.* (2014) found that partly coated sodium butyrate in the broiler diet significantly boosted feed intake, weight gain, and improved FCR. Dietary sodium butyrate induced weight gain and FCR up to 28 days of age, according to Mansoub (2011). Protected sodium butyrate, according to Pires *et al.*, (2020), improves the thickness, strength, and percentage of egg weight that may be attributed to the shell in aged laying hens' eggshells. Supplemental PSB lowers the percentages of broken and unclean eggs on a commercial level. Likewise, FCR and weight gain were increased by butyric acid (Panda *et al.*, 2009). Similarly, broiler performance during the grower and finisher stages was positively impacted by partially protected and microencapsulated sodium butyrate (Mallo *et al.*, 2010; Zou *et al.*, 2010a). Hernandez *et al.*, (2013) discovered that broiler flocks in commercial settings responded significantly to coated and uncoated sodium butyrate in terms of weight gain and FCR. The enhancement in broiler performance is considered due to different functions accomplished by sodium butyrate. In the small intestine, butyric acid lengthens the villi. In yellow-feathered breeder hens, coated SB was observed to decrease the F/E ratio while increasing the laying rate and daily egg weight (Wang *et al.*, 2021). Follicle-stimulating hormone secretion was induced, follicle growth and development were stimulated, and the laying rate was raised, according to Ghosh and Cox (1977). Additionally, CSB supplementation raised the laying ducks' ADFI and F/E ratio. According to other research, broiler chicken growth performance did not change when SB was supplemented at increasing doses of 500, 1000, or 2000 mg/kg (Wu *et al.*, 2018; Shareef *et al.*, 2017). According to other research, broiler starting period BW, FCR, and BWG were unaffected by sodium butyare (Letlole *et al.*, 2021). Additionally, Hanim *et al.* (2023) observed that broiler supplied with SB had higher body weight and average daily gain on day 35 when compared to the control group; additionally, liver weight, jejunum length, and colon length were raised with PSB supplementation, while heart weight was decreased on day 21.

Effect of Sodium Butyrate on Gut Health

Because of their long villi and shallow crypts, which offer a greater surface area for food absorption and a low rate of renewal, the intestinal cells can mature and produce enzymes more efficiently (Yang *et al.,* 2009). The morphology of broiler chickens' gastrointestinal tracts can be changed by any changes to their diet and gut microbiota. Each villus may extend or shorten in response to food changes in the bird's gut, which further influences nutrient absorption and digestion (Yang *et al.,* 2007). Research has shown that releasing products like SB into the small intestine early can improve nutritional digestibility and promote the growth of villus, while releasing them later into the cecum can limit the growth of gut pathogenic bacteria. The intestinal villus is essential for nutrition absorption and digestion (Awad *et al.,* 2015). The villus height and the region of interaction with the nutrients are correlated. Greater villus height enhances villus function, which in turn leads to improved bird growth performance. It was found in numerous earlier investigations that SB increased the height of the villus in the duodenum, jejunum, and ileum, the regions of the gut. According to Elnesr *et al.* (2019), butyrate enhances intestinal blood flow and gastrointestinal hormone production, which may be the reason behind SB's impact in improving intestinal condition. Moreover, BA causes an increase in peptide release, which boosts enterocyte proliferation and improves mucosa damage healing while also raising villi in height. Enterocytes preferentially absorb sodium butyrate as a source of energy because it is transformed to butyric acid after consumption (Mahdavi and Torki, 2009). It causes deeper crypts and taller villi by quickening the proliferation of enterocytes and villus elongation. According to studies, eating sodium butyrate (fat-coated food) caused an increase in villus height in the jejunum and ileum, but it had no effect on crypt depth or the ratio of villus height to crypt depth (Chamba *et al.,* 2014). According to Adil *et al.* (2011), there was a significantly greater response in terms of duodenal villi density to 3% sodium butyrate compared to 2% sodium butyrate. Dietary butyric acid (3% application rate) was found by Adil *et al.,* (2010) to considerably raise the height of villus in the duodenum and jejunum alone. Likewise, numerous studies have documented the advantageous impact of dietary sodium butyrate on broiler villi height and crypt depth throughout various stages of their development (Antongiovanni *et al.*, 2007; Mallo *et al.,* 2012). In broiler chickens treated with sodium butyrate, there was a decrease in the quantity of crypts in the jejunum and an increase in the height of the villi in the ileum (Hanim *et al.*, 2023)

Effect of Sodium Butyrate on Intestinal Bacterial Populations

Birds' intestines contain potentially harmful bacteria (such as *Salmonella, Clostridium* spp., or *Escherichia coli*) as well as health-promoting microorganisms (such as bifidobacteria or gram-positive lactobacilli). Typically, beneficial bacteria account for at least 85% of all bacteria. Due to its significant function in regulating the population of pathogenic bacteria and promoting the growth of beneficial bacteria in the bird's gut, SB has antibacterial properties. Due to its ability to reduce harmful microorganisms, adding SB to poultry diets can improve their health. According to Abdulqader and Al-Fataftah (2016), BA increased the viable counts of *Bifidobacterium* and *Lactobacillus.* Timbermont (2010) noted that SB has a positive impact on the management of necrotic enteritis. Additionally, adding SB to broilers' initial feed decreased the number of cases of Salmonella Enteritidis infections by day 27 (Fernandez-Rubio *et al.,* 2009). Because it lowers the pH of the gizzard, crop, and upper intestine while suppressing dangerous bacteria like *Salmonella spp., Escherichia coli,* and *Campylobacter jejuni,* sodium butyrate is a selective bactericidal agent (Van Deun *et al.,* 2008).

In contrast to diets supplemented with antibiotics, Chamba *et al.* (2014) did not report any impact of dietary sodium butyrate on E. coli populations in the jejunum. Similarly, Hu and Guo (2007) found that *E. coli* populations in the jejunum did not alter in response to varying amounts of sodium butyrate in diet. Similarly, compared to propionic acid, acetic acid, and L-lactate, coated butyric acid was found to be the most effective bactericidal agent against *Campylobacter jejuni* in vitro (Van Deun *et al.,* 2008). A larger dose of sodium butyrate in vitro had the same effect when intestinal mucus was present; however, feeding supplements containing sodium butyrate did not work against *C. jejuni* (Van Deun *et al.,* 2008). This suggested that in order to effectively combat *C. jejuni,* larger dosages of sodium butyrate might be required. According to a different study (Van Immerseel *et al.*, 2004), sodium butyrate inhibited the invasion of Salmonella enterica in the intestinal epithelium of broilers by downregulating *S. enterica's* pathogenicity island 1 (SPI1; Gantois *et al.,* 2006).

Conclusion

In summary, broiler and layer chickens can perform better in terms of growth, productivity, and gastrointestinal health by including dietary coated sodium butyrate in their diet.

9

Recent Advances in Management of Poultry Diseases

Gautham Kolluri, A.K. Tiwari, Shiva Kumar and Sai Siva Kumar

Avian Medicine Section, ICAR-Central Avian Research Institute Izatnagar-243122, Uttar Pradesh

Poultry production in India has emerged as a rapid growing sector among agricultural and livestock sector. Indian poultry industry has made a significant impact in economic, nutritional and socio-cultural aspects including livelihoods of poor rural households. Ever since its inception and is presently emerging as sun rise sector with a growth rate of 10-15% and overall turnover of Rs 70,000/- crore. Despite of frequent ingress with various pathogenic avian diseases including avian influenza, which is a severe setback for the industry, India has sustained globally as 3rd and 5th biggest country for egg and meat production respectively. Emerging and re-emerging poultry diseases in the country are posing significant challenges to the poultry industry. In the recent past, this sector has faced frequent onslaught of newer poultry diseases like bird flu (Avian Influenza) leading to enormous losses to the poultry sector not only in India but globally. In addition to this, other existing diseases viz. infectious bronchitis, infectious bursal disease, Ranikhet disease, Marek's disease and fowl pox have emerged in more virulent form. Therefore, scientific interventions are urgently needed to curb the menace of such emerging poultry diseases in the Country as well as effective control measures against already existing major poultry diseases.

The scenario of diseases has been changing frequently with a vast impact on poultry industry. Respiratory disease complex is emerged as a greatest challenge with multiple etiological pathogens. The existence of Infectious laryngotracheitis (ILT) in India was dated back to 1964, phylogenetic analysis in India revealed a close relatedness to vaccine strains. Infectious bronchitis also affected several Indian flocks with its ubiquitous existence. Mass, 793B

(4/91) and THA280252 are the important pathogenic strains that are commonly reported in the country. GHV Marek's disease, a lymphoproliferative disease of chickens is a great concern to poultry industry. The virus is shifting towards a more pathogenic trend with a striking emergence from mild to very virulent (vv) and very virulent plus (vv+). This developed a new clinical picture characterized by more than 90% morbidity and mortality and absence of classical signs, the lymphomas and peripheral neuritis while showing acute rashes. Recent epidemiological reports from India indicated high prevalence rate of 86% (serological) and 73.3% (molecular) for chicken infectious anaemia (CIA), vertically transmitted immunosuppressive disease of chicken. Phylogenetic analysis indicated a possibility of contaminated vaccines or infected breeders. Infectious bursal disease is found in Indian poultry flocks and continues to be as economic hardship for farmers. Contagious nature of virus coupled with geographically limited antigenic drift is always challenging since it is not possible to produce vaccine for every new strain encountered. Non-viral pathogenic agents Mycoplasma and *E. coli* are posing significant threats to the industry in form of secondary infections with frequent occurrence.

Does the Existing Conventional Disease Control Strategies are Insufficient?

Despite the vigorous growth and development, industry is facing challenges of emerging and new emerging diseases especially of viral origin with the periodical evolvement of more virulent strains. This continues to pose a serious threat to poultry production and the development of more effective coping strategies remains a significant challenge all the time. Possible sources of contamination inside the farm are the introduction of equipment from another farm; Feed and chick delivery vehicles, vehicles for lifting of farm birds; improper disposal of used litter; visitors, interchanging of farm personnel within the farm, veterinarians, company personnel; improper litter, manure and carcass disposal; backyard poultry, wild birds, rodents and other wild activity. Opened water sources nearby farms; replacement of birds; the introduction of chicks from contaminated hatcheries; contaminated vaccines, feed and water. Understanding the potential sources of infection in a farm is essential to deploy its curtailing measures. Accordingly, operations (Martin, 2016) should focus on establishing three disease barriers on their farm: *Physical barrier:* keeping disease and its vectors from making contact with the animals. All these operations must aim to minimize the risk of introduction of disease or contaminants by contractors, suppliers, visitors, company & health care personnel, personal movements, rodents, and vermin. *Chemical barrier:* killing the disease whenever possible by way of sanitation, and *Logical barrier:* ensuring farmers establish the correct management processes to minimize disease risk. The present paper mainly aims towards understanding of occurrence pattern of important viral diseases at national and global level in the light of control.

Housing and Ventilation

Sustained and apposite bio security and managmental (specially litter and droppings) practices must be employed from time and time. Farm management is of particular importance and things to look at include biosecurity, hygiene, environment and equipment, water quality and managing the brooding period. Even in all in-all out production system is used, elimination of any virus from a contaminated farm is little ambitious project and it is reasonable to aim at reducing the amount of virus present in the farm and consequently the amount of virus that challenge the chickens. Another key area of attention is health management including health and disease status and chick quality. An important part of the health issues in broilers originates from early infections with Enterobacteriaceae, staphylococci and enterococci with *E. cecorum* being the common. These infections are suggested to take place early in life, for example at the hatchery or shortly after placement on the farm. A different approach towards the hatching and brooding phase is the concept of on-farm hatching, currently available in two different systems: a multi-tier housing system, named Patio, and a system which is suitable for floor houses, named Xreck (Vencomatic Group, The Netherlands). Using these systems, broiler chickens are hatched inside the broiler house where they have direct access to feed and water and will remain during rest of the life. The conditions during the hatching and brooding phase in on-farm hatching systems largely differ from conditions in the hatchery, such as air temperature, relative humidity, air velocity, CO_2 level, dust level, disinfectant level, air volume per egg, chick handling, and transportation.

Minimum ventilation plays an important role in disease prevention inside the house by maintaining optimum air flow. This is the minimum amount of ventilation (air volume) required to maintain full genetic potential by ensuring an adequate supply of oxygen while removing the waster products of growth and combustion from the environment. Whenever the air quality begins to deteriorate there must be run time added to the 'on time and the 'off time' reduced to maintain the same total cycle length, because to add 'off time' as well, the percentage of run time would not change and the air quality results will not be improved.

As production modifications are mandated, new feeding and health challenges become more prevalent, i.e., difficulties maintaining feed consumption, monitoring supplementary nutrient intake and formulating a higher-energy diet. One of the most important feeding challenges posed by new animal welfare-focused production is to ensure adapted diets fulfill the metabolic needs and guarantee profitability to the farmer. Although, the impact on feed intake and performance may not always be substantial (new housing system) give rise to other concerns that could affect bird health and productivity-such as ammonia, emissions from the manure, risks of bone fractures due to flying, higher risks for diseases.

Feed Managemental Issues

Key points in feed formulation are limiting crude protein with optimization of digestible amino acids, encouraging gut development especially in terms of motility and acidification and the use of pre-starter to get the best possible start. Air and people flow should not provide opportunities for recontamination of treated feeds. Dust is a major source of salmonella contamination in feed mills and should be features in any monitoring programme. Alteration of physical form of diets: Lowering the grinding intensity of cereals in compound feeds or including a share of native/intact cereals in poultry diets is recommended for optimal gastrointestinal health. This not only avoids pro-ventricular dilatation in broilers, but also promotes desired effects on the microflora. There is one interesting fact that was neglected repeatedly in the past: the higher grinding intensity results in higher energy costs, but not conclusively in higher digestibility rates. Already a moderate grinding intensity guarantees 'normal' digestibility rates. Comparing studies in which different dietary particle size distributions were used, it can be concluded that a lower grinding intensity of cereals in diets for pigs and poultry without risks for reducing the digestibility rates is possible; with corn perhaps being one exception to this. Utilization of algae in poultry feeds currently being given more importance, as algae is proved to be efficient for mycotoxins control in feed via absorption. However, monitoring is important as algae also efficient in absorbing heavy metals and dioxins.

Feeding of Insects (Concept of Entomophagy)

Insects are also well known as an attractive and important natural source of food for many kinds of animals, including birds, lizards, snakes, amphibians, fish, insectivore, and other mammals. Insects generally have higher food conversion efficiency than other higher animals. Insects provide promising nutritional value to poultry diets and maximize ecological benefits with their edible nature. This makes insect meat more ecological than vertebrate's. Consumption of insects imparts a special flavour to poultry meat due to break down of amines during cooking. Also imparts yolk colour and taste to eggs produced.

These creatures have higher protein content ranging from 10-76% which depends on type of insect and developmental stage. Besides, they also possess good content of energy, high monounsaturated and/or polyunsaturated fatty acids, and are rich in micronutrients such as copper, iron, magnesium, manganese, phosphorous, selenium and zinc, as well as riboflavin, pantothenic acid, biotin and in some cases, folic acid. Protein production from insects for poultry consumption would be more effective and consume fewer resources than vertebrate/vegetable protein. Cereal proteins that are key staples in diets around the world are often low in lysine and in some cases, lack the amino acids tryptophan (e.g. maize) and threonine. Some reflects high amino acid content. Several caterpillars, palm weevil larvae and aquatic insects have amino acid scores for lysine higher than 100 mg amino acid per 100 g crude protein. Insects contain significant amounts of fibre, as measured by crude fibre, acid detergent fibre and neutral detergent fibre. The most common form of fibre in insects is chitin, an insoluble fibre derived from the exoskeleton. Chitin contains 7% Nitrogen (equivalent to 42% crude protein) and this is not readily digested by many. However, it is thought that, insectivorous birds including poultry possess chitinase enzyme required for its digestion. Chitin is associated with defense against parasitic infections and some allergic conditions.

In poultry, feed based on maggots, like larvae of black soldier fly (*Hermetia illucens*) is an attractive option to substitute current ingredients which are expensive and often in direct or indirect competition with human food. Some of the commonly available insect species for poultry in the country includes grasshoppers, black soldier fly, dragon flies, crickets, termites, ants, beetle larvae, moth caterpillars and pupae, giant water bugs, fleas, bees, wasps, earthworms cockroaches etc.

They are reported to have

Approximate composition of various insects meant for poultry feeding

Insect	Energy (Kcal)	Protein (g)	Iron (mg)	Thiamine (mg)	Riboflavin (mg)	Niacin (mg)
Termites	613	14.2	0.75	0.13	1.15	0.95
Caterpillar	370	28.2	35.5	3.67	1.91	5.2
Weevil	562	6.7	13.1	3.02	2.24	7.8

Composition of processed insect meals (Ravindran and Blair, 1993)

Content (%)	House fly Larvae meal	House fly Pupae meal	Silkworm Pupae meal	Grasshopper meal	Cricket meal	Earthworm meal
Crude protein	60	63	48	76	58	68
Crude fat	19	15	27	8	16	9
Crude fiber			3	9	9	3
Calcium	1	1	1			0.5
Phosphorus	3	8	1			0.8
Metabolizable energy (kcal/g DM)		2.5	2.9	2.7		2.4
Leucine	5.7	5.4	6.9	5.6	8.6	6.4
Isoleucine	3.1	3.6	4.0	2.9	5.3	5.2
Lysine	5.9	5.8	6.8	5.8	6.2	7.2
Methionine	2.3	2.6	2.9	1	1.3	2.0

Housefly provides viable option in poultry production. Feeding of magmeal made from housefly is found to be more economical. Maggots are readily available and are accredited for its high protein content with biological value exceeding that of soybean and groundnut. It possesses good amino acid profile, fats, metabolizable energy, minerals contents, fatty acid and is highly digestible than soybean meal.

The muscoid (Diptera) larvae and pupae from poultry manure or other organic wastes are used as a high protein source for broiler production. Dried house fly larvae, pupa contains high amount of protein (63.1%) and fat (15.5%) while 55.6 % crude protein and 5470 ME Kcal/Kg is present in maggot meal and can make up to 7% replacement for fish meal in broiler production without compromising production and sensory attributes of meat. Dried fly pupae can substitute soybean in chick diet up to 4 weeks of age. In addition, the short life of maggots and their production in large biomass from materials provide viable solution for manure management.

Larvae or pupae used to recycle nutrients from poultry manure or other organic wastes like cattle and swine manure, when these wastes used as a substrates for maggot production. Several methodologies including light induction have been developed for harvesting fly pupae from animal wastes. Silk worm pupae obtained from silk industry contains 48% protein and 27% crude fat with high vitamin content. Deoiled silk worm meal contains around 80% protein. It is observed that this can replace 50 and 100% of fish meal in brooder and layer mash diets respectively. High vitamin content, presence of unidentified production factor and ecdysteroids (hormone involved in metamorphosis) can improve fertility, hatchability, and production performance.

The use of insects particularly locust and grasshopper as poultry diets have been a great significance not only from the nutritional value, but also controlling pests. In one or other way reduces pesticide usage in agriculture, as these insects are mainly directed towards consumption. Besides insects other animal protein sources that can be utilized are snail and earth worm meal. Snail meal is rich nutrient source with 60% protein, 2% calcium, 0-8% phosphorus and 4% lysine. Boiled snail meal can replace up to 15% of maize in poultry diets.

Earthworms offer natural protein source for free range and scavenging poultry. One kg of earthworm biomass that has been obtained in $25m^2$ area can cater 15 birds for protein source replacing fish meal in chick and layer diets. Earthworm diets are known to reduce cholesterol content of eggs. Calcium and phosphorus supplementation is necessary since they have lower content of these due to absence of exoskeleton. Similarly, a soldier fly larva which is grown on cattle manure contains 42% crude protein and 35% fat. The European Commission (EC) has recently approved the use of processed animal proteins obtained from insects in aquafeeds (Regulation 2017/893/EC, 2017), and the Commission is currently working on authorizing their use in poultry feeds. Black soldier fly (*Hermetia illucens L*) could replace conventional poultry feed ingredients, such as soybean meal, which have a high environmental impact. HI larvae can provide high-value feedstuffs as they are rich in protein (37% to 63%) and have a better amino acid (AA) profile than soybean meal. Recent proximate analysis of black soldier fly revealed the following nutrient composition.

Crude protein; 42.04%; Crude fat: 42.04%; Nitrogen free extract: 9.21%; Calcium: 0.86%; Phosphorus: 0.3%; Dry matter: 98.43%; Organic matter: 79.4%;

Digestible amino acids: Methionine: 0.65%; Lysine: 1.43%; Cysteine: 0.18%; Isolecine: 1.6%; Leucine: 0.05%; Phenylalanine: 2.08%; Threonine: 1.24%; Tryptophan: 0.54%; Valine: 2.13%; Arginine: 3.44%.

Recent Experience

Following the COVID-19 attack in 2020, neighboring Pakistan and Rajasthan of India have been affected with severe locust swarm that destroyed the agriculture. This was then dealt with an idea of converting these threats to potential protein source for chicken and monogastrics (swine).

Establishment of Proper Gut Health

Optimizing gut health must be the prime most focus in poultry (broilers especially) to avoid future disease risk. While proper diet formulation is a major concern, disease prevention and immune support in a reduced or antibiotic free production scheme. Producers are faced with the challenge to exclude antibiotics while maintaining productive parameters to allow for the farm's profitability. Therefore, the formulation of diets for their specific effect on gut health is becoming a reality in the monogastric animal industries. The maintenance of gut health is essential when antibiotics are not used. With 70% of animal's immunity concentrated in the gut, fostering a strong gastrointestinal system will improve its health, performance and welfare. Everything in the gastrointestinal tract is connected: the nutrition, the microbiome and gut and immune function. Supplementation of protease with adaptive direct-fed-microbial improves barrier strength through tight junctions, enhance protein digestibility, amino acid utilization and fiber-bound nutrient release.

Lessening the time gap between the hatch and first exposure to feed in chick life is essential for the development of intestinal tract and so better able to resist any disease challenges in later life. Monitoring and evaluation of intestinal integrity index (I2). The generated I^2 score reflects the daily weight gain, FE and allows any changes in poultry health protocols. Integrating organic acids with pre and probiotics will help to reduce the gut thickness, establishing and stabilizing normal microbiota would increases gut absorptive and digestive functionalities.

Mitigating anti-microbial resistance by precisely following the recommended dosage of sub-therapeutic antibiotics has increased over last 60 years, from 10-20 g/ton in the early 1950s to 40-50 g/ton in the 1970s to 30-110 g/ton nowadays. Replacing AGPs relies upon a holistic approach to improve animal health status and performance through better management, bio-security, vaccination, diagnostics and feeding strategy. α-monoglycerides such as α-monoproionin and α-monobutyrin are reported to have potential antibacterial actions that can be used to replace antibiotic growth promoters confidently.

Mono-glyceride derivatives of lauric acid i.e., α-monolaurin hahve antiviral properties. These ingredients are active in the entire gastro-intestinal tract. Depending on the chain length of the fatty acid, they are active against gram negative or gram-positive bacteria and against fat enveloped viruses.

Micro-encapsulation concept has been integrated in delivering the phytogenic active compounds and essential oils ensures sustained release of substances over a period of time and yields a stabilized biological action. They reported to have appetising and endogenous secretions, gut microbiota modulation, gut protection.

Electrolyzed oxidizing water (Nontox) provides a real alternative to formaldehyde. This is the result of electro-chemical activation of salt and water. The disinfecting action comes from free radicals in combination with active chlorine compounds such as HClO and ClO. This reported to leave no residues on the surface of hatchery with no buildup of bacterial resistance.

Vaccines, Vaccination and Its Impact

The successful control strategy mainly lies in the wisdom of identifying new variants associated with disease in vaccinated birds along with in time characterization of pathogenicity of new virus variant. Preference for good vaccine brand, choice is important as some vaccines show lower replication rates leading to delayed and/or weak immunity; Adoption of Intelligent vaccine handling and vaccine administration practices. Focus on new technology vaccines may drive disease control strategies towards a safe line. These include immune complex vaccines, vector HVT vaccines and vector FP vaccines. Most commonly they exclusively based once vector HVT technology. ''HVT plus IBDV-VP2'' vector vaccines have been developed for application in-ovo or by the subcutaneous route in 1-day-old chickens and has also been licensed in various countries (Le Gros*et al.*, 2009). It is also proved to have remarkable effect on variant IBDV (Perozo *et al.*, 2009). IBDV immune complex vaccines consisting of IBDV-specific antibodies obtained from the sera of hyperimmunized chickens and infectious IBD vaccine virus have showed better protection against live vaccines when given subcutaneously (Muller *et al.*, 2012). New technology vaccines are becoming popular with global usage of 45% in the hatchery. Amongst the three targeted major diseases, new technology vaccines against IBD are the front runners, which were the first to be introduced (from 2002 to 2008) and have the largest usage share followed by ND new technology vaccines, whose percentage is rapidly expanding (Comte, 2013). Further, changing towards an efficient vaccine technology with continuous cell lines other that CEFs minimize the number of aseptic handlings during production and increase the possibility for production in bioreactors. Vaccines currently available are Tissue culture origin (TCO), Chicken Embryo Origin (CEO) and Recombinant fowl pox vaccines. Flock coverage in ILT is critical, as vaccine virus spreads rapidly and cause disease in non-vaccinated birds (Fulton *et al.*, 2000). Among these, CEO vaccines even though can be applied with ease in field by mass vaccination, they may have potential to increase their virulence with bird-to bird passage. In the line of improving vaccine efficacy, stringent laws may be imposed on vaccine usages and their marketing pattern.

Because of limited and short-lasting efficacy of live and killed vaccines applied in the presence of MDA, boosting vaccinations are necessary and in many countries can even be considered as the backbone of diseases protection. Depending upon the perception of infectious pressure 1,2 or more boosting vaccinations can be employed in broilers before slaughter and in pullets, this number is increased up to 3-5 before transfer. Live vaccination efficiency is solely depending upon the way it is being administered. In parent stocks, protection during laying is assured by injection of killed/inactivated vaccines at the point of lay or just before the lay. The protective efficacy depends on antigenic load and timing of previous priming with live vaccines.

Maternally derived antibodies (MDA) are extremely effective in protecting young chickens against diseases during first few weeks of life and therefore it is to ensure their high and homogenous population with intelligent vaccination protocols. Vaccination efficiency for IBD extremely depends upon the MDA titer and by employing the Deventer's formula, the optimal age of a chick for IBD vaccination can be determined as follows

$$\{(\log_2 \text{titre bird\%} - \log_2 \text{breakthrough}) \times t_{1/2}\} + \text{age at sampling} + \text{correction 0-4}$$

Key challenges for effective AI vaccination include, ensuring post vaccination virus surveillance and sero-monitoring; vaccinating the birds with a strain that is matching with circulating field strains; Managing effective public-private partnerships, financial sustainability, and producing field-based evidence for making decisions, particularly in relation to investigating the reasons for vaccine failure (FAO, 2011). The main snag with the avian influenza vaccination is that majority of virus outbreaks in poultry may be hidden as LPAI infections and vaccinated birds can be sub clinically infected upon exposure to field virus (Berry, 2013). Vaccination may be complemented with control strategies were stamping out technique alone is ineffective (Lee and Suarez, 2006).

Monitoring of Pathogens Spread

Continuous monitoring of potential spread of unique genotypes by predicting global movement of poultry and poultry products. In this line, use of geographic information system (GIS) technology is beneficial. In poultry, GIS technology is an ideal tool for disease surveillance, outbreak control and emergency management (Johnson *et al.*, 2000). It has served many poultry related issues for the last ten years in many countries. GIS technology allows for accurate location of all premises, quick adjustments of any changes in the data and manipulation and analysis of the data for sound decision-making besides providing a base for design of vaccination zones and demarcation between vaccinated and non-vaccinated zones. Further grid and road maps even though pose little difficulty, when all the farms are mapped, provides an information of not only affected farm but also the susceptible premises around them, which is difficult to achieve with other maps. Computer software is used to draw zones of biosecurity or vaccination during an outbreak (Dofour, 2008). Studying genetic variation within populations of viruses that includes their geographic distribution (Phylogeography) allows tracking of spatial diffusion process for a virus as it occurs over time and mostly for highly contagious diseases like IBDV.

Disease Prediction

Implementation of surveillance programmes in commercial poultry facilities to detect AI virus infections and includes **Syndromic surveillance** for the early detection of notifiable AI by clinical symptoms specific to mainly HPAI subtypes but not LPAI; **Early warning surveillance** for exclusion diagnostics. Birds showing clinical signs pathognomonic for infection with pathogens other than AI cannot be excluded; **Serological monitoring** programme to detect all AI virus incursions even the non-notifiable ones and those that remain subclinical.

Attempts must be made to arrive at advanced standard platforms like biosensors, nano-molecules for on farm disease diagnosis in time. To added this, a new portable biosensor based H5N1 detection system in field has been developed and in the way of its field trials. It was observed that, this unit could detect virus in poultry samples within an hour. Bio-aerosol sampling for the avian influenza virus detection is the recently budding technique and introduced recently by the threat prompted researchers, of IGHI, introduced aerosol sampling for avian influenza viruses in Vietnam for increased accuracy of diagnosis. The aerosol tripods are employed at 0.5 m from cages and 0.2-1.5 m from live birds. Quantitative reverse-transcription polymerase chain reaction results revealed a 92% positive correlation with oro-pharyngeal swabs.

Focus on Disease Resistance

Focus on developing disease resistant chicken lines through immune genetics and transgenics mediated approaches by exploiting the hidden innate immune mechanisms of alternate poultry species like Ducks and Guinea fowl which showed to have stronger immune competence traits against most common poultry diseases. Similarly, revealing the mechanisms responsible for harboring the influenza virus in wild birds, water fowls, migratory birds and house crow should be the utmost priority.

10

Plant-based Edible Vaccines for Poultry: Promises, Challenges and Future Prospects

Vasanthi Balan

Assistant Professor, Poultry Research Station, Tamil Nadu Veterinary and Animal Sciences University (TANUVAS), Madhavaram Milk Colony Chennai – 600 051, Tamil Nadu

A novel approach to immunisation is edible vaccines that work by using plants as bio factories to create immunogenic proteins that, when ingested, can provide immunity. The idea is to genetically modify plants such that they express genes that code for pathogen proteins or antigens. Then, because they stimulate the synthesis of vaccine components within their tissues, these genetically engineered plants serve as vaccine delivery vehicles. The hepatitis B vaccination served as the model for immunogenicity in humans in the early research on edible vaccines. The development of edible vaccines is still the subject of extensive research conducted internationally, and the findings are positive in terms of avoiding infectious diseases in animals as well humans.

Mechanism of Production of Edible Vaccines

1. **Genetic Modification (Introduction of Genes):** Specific genes encoding antigens or immunogenic proteins are introduced into the genome of plants.
2. **Transgenic Plants (Expression of Proteins):** The transgenic plants express and produce the desired immunogenic proteins within their tissues.
3. **Oral Administration (Consumption by Poultry):** Poultry consumes the transgenic plants containing the immunogenic proteins.

4. **Immune Response Activation (Stimulation of Immunity):** The ingested proteins stimulate both mucosal and systemic immune responses in poultry.
5. **Protection Against Diseases (Specific Immunity):** The activated immune response provides protection against specific poultry diseases targeted by the edible vaccine.

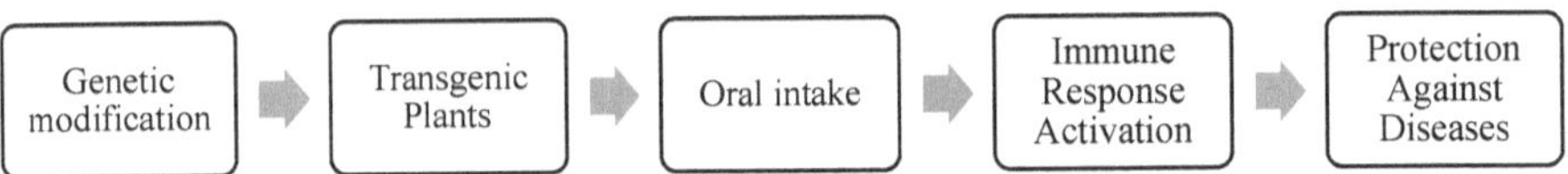

Fig. Mechanism of production of plant-based edible vaccines

Production of poultry plant- based edible vaccines

A complex approach combining plant biology and genetic engineering is used to produce palatable vaccines for poultry. The technique consists of multiple crucial steps that eventually lead to the creation of transgenic plants that can produce immunogenic proteins for oral vaccination.

Key steps in production of plant- based edible vaccines

1. Selection of Antigens (Identification of target diseases)

The process of selecting antigens (or immunogenic proteins) unique to the poultry diseases of interest involves identifying the target diseases.

2. Genetic Modification (Introduction of genes)

Specific genes encoding the identified antigens are introduced into the genome of plants. This is typically achieved through techniques such as Agrobacterium-mediated transformation.

3. Transgenic Plant Development (Gene expression)

The transgenic plants express the introduced genes, leading to the synthesis and accumulation of the desired immunogenic proteins within their tissues. Once the transgenic plants are induced to manufacture the encoded proteins, they effectively become bio factories for vaccine production. The plant tissues, such as leaves or seeds, serve as the source of the edible vaccine.

4. Cultivation and Harvesting (Optimized growth conditions)

Transgenic plants are cultivated under controlled conditions to optimize the expression of immunogenic proteins. Plant parts with the highest concentration of immunogenic proteins, such as leaves or seeds, are harvested.

5. Processing and Formulation

a. **Extraction and Purification:** Immunogenic proteins are extracted from the harvested plant material and purified to ensure their effectiveness.

b. **Formulation:** The purified proteins are formulated to create the final edible vaccine product.

6. Packaging and Distribution

The edible vaccines are packaged into suitable forms for administration, such as feed or plant material and the formulated edible vaccine is distributed to poultry farms for oral administration.

7. Oral Administration and immune response activation

Edible vaccines are designed to be consumed orally. Poultry consumes the transgenic plants or formulated feed containing the immunogenic proteins and the ingested immunogenic proteins stimulate both mucosal and systemic immune responses in poultry, conferring protection against specific diseases.

Advantages of plant-based edible vaccines in poultry farming

Plant-based edible vaccines play a crucial role in poultry farming, offering several significant advantages over traditional vaccination methods and contributes to advancements in disease prevention and sustainable farm practices. These advantages include:

1. Convenient administration of oral vaccination

Plant-based edible vaccines enable oral vaccination, eliminating the need for injections. This simplifies the vaccination process in poultry farming, reducing stress on birds and the labour and equipment requirement associated with traditional vaccination methods. This ease of administration provides a convenient and cost-effective alternative, especially in resource-limited settings.

2. Cost-effectiveness and scalability of production

The use of plants as bio factories for vaccine production is cost-effective. Edible vaccines provide an economically viable alternative, particularly in regions where cost constraints may limit the widespread adoption of traditional vaccines. Plant-based vaccines are relatively easier and less expensive to manufacture, in contrast to traditional vaccine production, which often requires sophisticated and expensive facilities contributing to their economic feasibility. It offers a cost-effective and scalable alternative to traditional vaccine production methods, particularly in resource-limited settings.

Further the production of edible vaccines, especially in plants, allows for scalability and rapid deployment. This agility is beneficial in responding to emerging infectious diseases or large-scale vaccination campaigns.

3. Targeted protection and disease prevention

Plant-based edible vaccines can be designed to provide protection against specific poultry diseases, such as Newcastle disease, Avian influenza or coccidiosis. This targeted approach enhances the effectiveness of disease prevention strategies in poultry farms.

4. Reduced environmental impact

Utilizing plants for vaccine production contributes to sustainable and environmentally friendly farming practices. Edible vaccines can reduce the reliance on conventional vaccine production methods, which may have environmental implications.

5. Minimizes risk of infection

Plant-based edible vaccines reduce the risk of contamination associated with traditional injection methods. This biosecurity benefit is especially crucial in preventing the spread of diseases within poultry flocks. Further by avoiding the use of needles, edible vaccines offer a needle-free immunization approach. This can help overcome needle-related challenges such as needle disposal issues, and the risk of needle-transmitted infections.

6. Enhanced immune response

Plant-based edible vaccines, when consumed, stimulate both mucosal and systemic immune responses in poultry. This dual response contributes to robust immunity, enhancing the overall health and well-being of the flock. Edible vaccines have shown promising results in terms of efficacy and immunogenicity, offering a novel approach to vaccination. Research indicates several key aspects highlighting their effectiveness. Plant-derived vaccines demonstrate immunogenicity, stimulating both systemic and mucosal immune responses in the host organisms. Edible vaccines trigger the production of specific antibodies, providing protection against targeted pathogens.

Further edible vaccines offer the advantage of long-lasting immunity without the possibility of relapse reactions.

7. Simplifies storage and logistics

The distribution and storage of these vaccines are more straightforward compared to traditional vaccines that often require refrigeration and careful handling. : Edible vaccines, especially those derived from plants, can be more stable at higher temperatures, reducing the dependency on a strict cold chain for storage and transportation. This characteristic is particularly advantageous in reaching remote or resource-limited poultry farms.

8. Customizable solutions and adaptability

Plant-based edible vaccines offer flexibility in designing vaccines tailored to the specific needs of poultry farms. This adaptability allows for the development of vaccines against a range of poultry diseases.

Hence the significance of plant-based edible vaccines in poultry farming lies in their ability to provide a cost-effective, convenient, and targeted approach to disease prevention. These vaccines contribute to sustainable farming practices while promoting the overall health and productivity of poultry flocks. Ongoing research in this field continues to enhance the efficacy and applicability of this innovative vaccination approach.

Applications of plant- based edible vaccines against poultry diseases:

Plant-based edible vaccines offer promising applications in combating poultry diseases. This innovative approach leverages plants as bio factories for producing antigens, which, when consumed by poultry, can induce an immune response. Oral immunization with transgenic plants expressing antigens relevant to poultry pathogens has been explored and have shown promise in addressing specific poultry diseases, offering a cost-effective and innovative approach. Notable examples include:

1. Protection against viral diseases

Plant-based edible vaccines have been studied for their efficacy against viral diseases in poultry. Oral immunization with these transgenic plants expressing viral antigens aims to confer protection against specific viral pathogens. Edible vaccines have been explored to address respiratory viral diseases like New castle disease, Avian influenza, that causes severe economic consequences. By expressing relevant antigens from viruses in plants, these vaccines aim to induce protective immunity when consumed by poultry. Similarly, Plant-based edible vaccines have also been investigated to express antigens related to Infectious bursal disease (IBD), contributing to disease prevention in a cost-effective manner.

2. Control of bacterial infections

The technology also holds potential for controlling bacterial infections in poultry. Edible vaccines expressing antigens related to bacterial pathogens could stimulate the chicken's immune system, providing a means of disease control.

3. Prevention of parasitic diseases

Plant-based vaccines have been developed to combat coccidiosis, a significant parasitic disease affecting poultry. These vaccines aim to express antigens related to coccidian parasites, providing an oral immunization method to control the disease.

These examples demonstrate the versatility of plant-based vaccines in addressing a range of poultry health challenges. Plant-based vaccines are characterized by their cost-effectiveness, thermostability, and absence of human or animal pathogens, making them a promising technology for poultry disease prevention.

Protective sfficacy studies of plant-based edible vaccines in poultry

Plant-based edible vaccines have shown to be effective against *Eimeria tenella*, a protozoan parasite affecting poultry. The vaccines were produced in tobacco leaves, and the immunogenic response was considerably high compared to control groups, indicating potential protection against this poultry pathogen.

Further in a study, it has been explored that the oral delivery of cytokines expressed in edible plants as vaccine adjuvants in chickens, marking a significant step in understanding the crosstalk between immunization and edible vaccines. These findings suggest that the expression of immunogenic proteins in plants, intended for use as edible vaccines, can influence the host's immune response, potentially involving proinflammatory pathways. However, further research is essential to comprehensively understand the implications and mechanisms underlying the production of proinflammatory cytokines in response to immunogenic protein expression.

Also, oral immunization with recombinant Lactobacillus plantarum has been explored as a novel vaccination strategy. In a study, chickens were orally immunized with a recombinant L. plantarum containing the gp85 protein. Gp85 is a protein associated with avian leukosis virus subgroup J (ALV-J). The research aimed to investigate the efficacy of this oral vaccine, and the results showed that chickens immunized with recombinant L. plantarum exhibited enhanced immune responses, including increased antibody levels, particularly IgA. Furthermore, the study indicated a potential in preventing body weight loss associated with ALV-J infection, suggesting the protective effects of the oral vaccine in chickens. This approach leverages the use of Lactobacillus plantarum as a live vector for delivering recombinant antigens, potentially offering a convenient and effective means of vaccination in poultry.

These studies collectively underscore the potential of plant-based edible vaccines for poultry in providing protection against a range of pathogens, including protozoa, viruses, bacteria, and parasites. Continued research in this field is essential to refine and optimize these vaccines for practical applications in poultry farming.

Limitations and challenges in plant-based edible vaccine development

Plant-based edible vaccines, while holding great promise, face certain limitations and challenges in their development:

1. **Immunotolerance Issues**: The subjects may develop immunotolerance to specific vaccine proteins, reducing the effectiveness of subsequent doses
2. **Dosage Control**: Achieving consistent dosage and expression of antigens in plants can be challenging, impacting the vaccine's efficacy and reproducibility
3. **Stability and Storage**: Maintaining the stability of vaccine antigens in edible form, especially in varying environmental conditions, poses a challenge
4. **Regulatory Approval**: Navigating complex regulatory processes and establishing safety and efficacy criteria are hurdles for widespread acceptance
5. **Consumer Acceptance**: Overcoming scepticism and ensuring consumer acceptance of edible vaccines, particularly in certain cultures, requires educational efforts
6. **Standardization:** Standardizing the expression of antigens in plant-based vaccines is essential for reliable and effective immunization

Future prospects

Plant-based edible poultry vaccines present both challenges and promising prospects in the field of poultry industry.

1. The potential for cost-effective production, make them accessible for poultry farmers and enhance disease prevention in poultry populations.
2. Further tailoring edible vaccines for specific poultry diseases, such as coccidiosis and avian influenza, can provide targeted and effective disease control strategies.
3. Developing plant-based edible vaccines with enhanced stability at

higher temperatures can reduce the dependency on a strict cold chain, facilitating easier distribution.

4. The scalability and rapid deployment capabilities of plant-based edible vaccines make them valuable tools in responding to disease outbreaks, allowing for quick and widespread immunization.

Further exploration and refinement of plant-based edible vaccines for poultry diseases, addressing challenges and enhancing their efficacy. Persistent efforts to develop plant-based vaccines targeting other economically important diseases like *Mycoplasma* in poultry helps to overcome challenges in their development.

Conclusion

In conclusion, plant-based poultry edible vaccines have proven to be effective in eliciting a strong immunogenic response, protecting against various viruses, bacteria, and parasitic diseases affecting poultry, including Avian influenza, Newcastle disease, and Coccidiosis, and offers practical advantages such as cost-effectiveness, ease of administration, long-lasting immunity, and potential for scalability, making plant-based vaccines a viable alternative for poultry immunization. Continued research and development in this field focuses on addressing various challenges and leveraging the advantages offered by this innovative approach and holds the potential to further optimize these vaccines for widespread use in poultry farming.

References

Natsumi Takeyama, Hiroshi Kiyono, and Yoshikazu Yuki (2015) Plant-based vaccines for animals and humans: recent advances in technology and clinical trials. Ther Adv Vaccines, 3 (1) : 139-154.

Aswathi P. B, Bhanja S, K, Yadav A, S, Rekha V, John J, K, Gopinath D, Sadanandan G,V, Shinde A, Jacob A (2014). Plant-based edible vaccines against poultry diseases: a review. Adv. Anim. Vet. Sci. 2 (5): 305 – 311.

Vrinda M Kurup and Jaya Thomas (2020) Edible Vaccines: Promises and Challenges, Mol Biotechnol, 62 (2): 79-90

11

CocciConundrum A Comprehensive Exploration of Conventional Strategies to Advance Insights for Poultry Coccidiosis

Vivek Agrawal[1], Girraj Goyal[2], Mukesh Shakya[1] and Nidhi Singh Choudhary[3]

[1]Department of Veterinary Parasitology, College of Veterinary Science & Animal Husbandry, Mhow (M.P.)
[2]Department of Poultry Science, College of Veterinary Science and Animal Husbandry, Jabalpur-482001 (M.P.)
[3]Department of Veterinary Medicine, College of Veterinary Science and Animal Husbandry, Mhow - 453445 (M.P.)

Losses caused by *Eimeria* in Intestine of poultry are well known from more than century (Chapman, 2014) and their important information like life cycle, pathogenesis, global distribution are well established (Shirley *et al.*, 2005). Heavy infection of coccidiosis in poultry leads to necrotic enteritis, reduced feed conversion ratio and even some species of *Eimeria* are responsible for mortality of birds (Shirley *et al.*, 2005; Williams, 1999). Due to economic losses caused by *Eimeria*, prophylactic use of anticoccidial drugs and live parasitic vaccine are used in poultry industry (Blake and Tomley, 2014).

Anticoocidial drug sensitivity test is only available method to diagnose the anticoccidial drug resistance (Naciri *et al.*, 2003) nevertheless it has so many inherent limitation like very expensive, collected oocyst are from outbreak of coccidiosis which are not true representative of sample further propagation in chicks lead to multiplication of non resistant *Eimeria* spp. also. Unlike the bacteria and virus in case of Eimeria no major studies has been occurred at molecular level due to complex structure and mechanism involved. Otherwise it is imperative to know the exact mechanism behind the development of resistance against anticoccidial drugs as well as against vaccine.

Allelic diversity of selected gene encoding antigens used to make recombinant vaccine play a seminal role if allelic diversity is more then chances of failure of vaccine is more due to immune escape (*Plasmodium falciparum* with the antimalarial vaccine candidates apical membrane antigen 1 (AMA1) and merozoite surface antigen 1 (MSP1) (Arnott *et al.*, 2014; Takala and Plowe, 2009) but on the other hand selection pressure on recombinant antigen is less. Due to low selection pressure the chances of development of resistance against recombinant vaccine is less.

Selection pressure on *Eimeria* is very high due to mainly peculiarity of parasite as well as host. The fecundity, replication of parasite and on the other end high number of host and their intense farming and rapid turnover are the major factor for high selection pressure. These are the determinants for the development of anticoccidial resistance (Chapman, 1997). In live vaccine, whole parasite are used which shows 6000-9000 antigens during their completion of life cycle (Reid *et al.*, 2014). Therefore till date even after the use of 50 years, no resistance has been reported against live vaccine but situation is different for recombinant vaccine because in it few antigens are used then there are more chances immune evasion or resistance by parasite might be occurred owing to more focused genetic selection pressure. Due to this limiting factor, commercial production of recombinant vaccine did not get desired pace.

Global Challenges: Antigenic Quests, Consumer and Safety Concerns

Coccidiosis caused by *Eimeria* protozoa belong to phylum Apicomplexa and it is very close relative of *Toxoplasma gondii* and *Plasmodium* spp. *Eimeria* is having capacity to infect all livestock but most of the species of *Eimeria* are host specific (Vrba and Pakandl, 2015). Coccidiosis causing heavy economic loss to poultry industry which is approximately £2 billion (Lassen and Ostergaard, 2012). There are seven species of *Eimeria* Viz; *Eimeria tenella*, *Eimeria necatrix* or *Eimeria brunetti*, and *Eimeria acervulina, Eimeria maxima, Eimeria mitis* or *Eimeria praecox* causing clinical coccidiosis manifested in form of haemorrhagic or malabsorptive enteritis (Williams *et al.*, 2009).

Broiler industry of poultry is bigger than layer or breeder industry (McDonald and Shirley, 2009) and live vaccine is not recommended for broiler due to some inherited problems like development of subclinical coccidiosis, hence there is dire requirement of recombinant vaccine for broiler sector as in some country like USA and European union there is ban on anticoccidial drugs due to residue of drug are harmful to consumers. Researcher and academia both are actively involved to find out golden bullet or cocktail of antigen against closely related parasite like *Toxoplasma gondii* and *Plasmodium* spp. but they did not get it owing to high standard (Gedik *et al.*, 2016). Same things might be happened with Eimeria spp. also.

Genetic Diversity and Plasticity: Unraveling the Mysteries of Ionophore Resistance

Leakiness pays a seminal role during use of ionophores and there are multifaceted advantage of that phenomena viz few *Eimeria* oocyst remain unexposed leads to development of immunity owing to trickle infection of Eimeria oocyst and there is low selection pressure on *Eimeria* oocyst which helps to slow development of resistance. Owing to a aforementioned rationale, ionophores are the anticoccidial drugs which share more than 70% of anticoccidial drug market globally (Eckford *et al.*, 2014), although due to health concern issue Codex put maximum residue limit of anticoccidial in meat and accordingly European union and United states have curtain the use of anticoccidial and encouraging the use of vaccine for control of economically significant coccidiosis. Nonetheless after introduction of ionophores, resistance against them documented might be due to pre exiting genetic diversity of *Eimeria* spp. or high genome plasticity.

Latest Advances in Vaccine Development

The concept of vaccine against *Eimeria* came in to existence when poultry become resistant to further infection of *Eimeria* after ingestion of homologous *Eimeria* spp. This was the basis for modern coccidiology vaccine. The first vaccine developed against *Eimeria* was live vaccine i.e. Coccivac. The inherent limitation of live vaccine was to develop the lesion in intestine and leading to subclinical coccidiosis. Another major constraint is cost of production (Blake and Tomley, 2014). These limitation resulted the development of attenuated vaccine which is having upper hands as far as the production of lesion is concerned which is absent in case of attenuated vaccine and their low cost of production (Chapman and Jeffers, 2014) but at the same time by using the attenuated vaccine(Paracox), we lost the brighter site of live vaccine that is reversal of susceptibility of anticoccidial drug against *Eimeria* (Chapman and Jeffers, 2015). In Europe live vaccine is not currently licenced due to their vaccine induced drawback. Production of both type of vaccine at mass level is major hindrance somewhere and immunity achieved during the attenuated vaccine was not up to desired level therefore there is need for the development of subunit vaccine.

The first subunit vaccine was CoxAbic used commercially at broad scale. It is based on gam56 and gam82 purified from gametocyte of *E. maxima.* It is vital antigen as it involved in synthesis of oocyst wall due to which it become resistant against adverse environmental condition and transmission of occyst occur very quickly. As there is protein cross linked via ditrypsin bond required during cell wall synthesis. It is documanted that provide the protection upto 8 week in broiler chick which is the age to sale in market. Another key feature of CoxAbic is that it provide the immunity against multiple species of *Eimeria* (Smith, 1994) unlike direct immunity which is species specific (Rose, 1987). But the in vivo production of parasitic antigen as well as requirement of boosting under field condition is limiting factors (Wallach, 2008). Lot of work has been done in that direction and it has been documented that apicalcomlex pay important role at the time of penetration of oocyst and Apical membrane antigen 1(AMA1) (Rugarabamu *et al.*,2015) used for production of recombinant vaccine. Rhomboid like protease involved in processing of MIC also used as recombinant protein and used as DNA or Myco-bacterium bovis vectored formulations (Wang *et al.*, 2014). Glycosyl-phosphatidylinositol (GPI) anchored surface antigen (SAG)1 which is encoded by multi gene families was also tried by various worker as it play important role at the site of attachment to the host prior to invasion(Song *et al.*, 2015). Immune mapped protein 1(IMP1) localized on sporozoite cell membrane also used as anticoccidial vaccine candidate for *E. maxima* and *E. tenella* (Yin *et al.*, 2015). Profiline is an actine biding protein and involved in microfilament turnover which play pivotal role in gliding moment of T. *gondii* (Plattner *et al.*, 2008) and also a ligand for toll like receptors 5, 11 and 12 which play important role for initiating the immune response against many intracellular pathogens. During the Eimeria infection up regulation of TLR has been reported (Zhang *et al.*, 2012).

Harnessing Cytokine Power: A Game-Changer in Recombinant Vaccines

Type and dose of cytokine affect the efficacy of recombinant antigens like IFNα and lymphotactin were found to improve weight gain during *E. acervulina* challenge, while IL-1β, IL-8, IL-15, IFNy, TGFb4 and lymphotactin decreased parasite replication. It has been documented that administration of IL-2 with Eimeria antigen such as TA4 (Song *et al.*, 2009;) SO7 (Song *et al.*, 2013) and *E. acervulina* antigen zSZ-2 (Shah *et al.*, 2011) can enhance the DNA vaccine induced protective immunity. By combining the CD40 ligand with IMP1, improvement of antigen presenting cell activation and downstream T-cell mediated effectors functions could be achieved (Yin *et al.*, 2015).

Vaccine Odyssey: Overcoming Eimeria's Genetic and Antigenic Maze

As per the available literature, there are lot of difference between different strain of *Eimeria* for example isolate of *E. tenella* from north India has low haploid while isolates from south India has high haploid (Blake *et al.*, 2015). It might be due to different managemental practices at both geographical regions. Likewise operational taxonomic unit viz. OTUx OTUy and OTUz have been reported worldwide (Godwin and Morgan 2015) with the help of advanced technology like Rstriction fragment length polymorphism (PCR-RFLP), Amplified fragment length polymorphism (AFLP) and Random amplified polymorphic DNA (RAPD) and variable number tandem repeat (VNTR) (Pegg *et al.* 2016). Similarly Apical membrane antigen gene are polymorphic and hence create major hindrance for development of recombinant vaccine using the AMA1.

Conclusion

Emergences of new variants among Eimeria parasite in different geographical area pose a major menace for the development of vaccine against coccidiosis. Therefore it is imperative to study the evolution of diversity among gene along with other associate factor for development of effective vaccine.

References

Arnott, A., Wapling, J., Mueller, I., Ramsland, P. A., Siba, P. M., Reeder, J. C., & Barry, A. E. (2014). Distinct patterns of diversity, population structure and evolution in the AMA1 genes of sympatric Plasmodium falciparum and Plasmodium vivax populations of Papua New Guinea from an area of similarly high transmission. Malaria Journal, 13(1), 1-16.

Blake, D. P., & Tomley, F. M. (2014). Securing poultry production from the ever-present Eimeria challenge. Trends in Parasitology, 30(1), 12-19.

Chapman, H. D. (1997). Biochemical, genetic and applied aspects of drug resistance in Eimeria parasites of the fowl. Avian Pathology, 26(2), 221-244.

Chapman, H.D. (2014). Milestones in avian coccidiosis research: a review. Poultry Science, 93(3), 501-511.

Chapman, H. D., & Jeffers, T. K. (2015). Restoration of sensitivity to salinomycin in Eimeria following 5 flocks of broiler chickens reared in floor-pens using drug programs and vaccination to control coccidiosis. Poultry Science, 94(5), 943-946.

Eckford, S., Grace, K., Harris, C., Reeves, H., Teale, C., Tallentire, C., 2014. UK-VARSS 2013. In: Borriello, S. (Ed.), UK Veterinary Antibiotic Resistance and Sales Surveillance Report.

Gedik, Y., İz, S. G., Can, H., Döşkaya, A. D., Gürhan, S. İ. D., Gürüz, Y., & Döşkaya, M. (2016). Immunogenic multistage recombinant protein vaccine confers partial protection against experimental toxoplasmosis mimicking natural infection in murine model. Trials in Vaccinology, 5, 15-23.

Godwin, R. M., & Morgan, J. A. (2015). A molecular survey of Eimeria in chickens across Australia. Veterinary Parasitology, 214(1-2), 16-21.

Lassen, B., & Østergaard, S. (2012). Estimation of the economical effects of Eimeria infections in Estonian dairy herds using a stochastic model. Preventive Veterinary Medicine, 106 (3-4), 258-265.

McDonald, V., & Shirley, M. W. (2009). Past and future: Vaccination against Eimeria. Parasitology, 136(12), 1477-1489.

Naciri, M., Chausse, A. M., Fort, G., Bernardet, N., Nerat, F., & de Gussem, K. (2004, June). Utility of anticoccidial sensitivity tests (ASTs) in the prevention of chicken coccidiosis. In 22. World's Poultry Congress. WPSA.

Pegg, E., Doyle, K., Clark, E. L., Jatau, I. D., Tomley, F. M., & Blake, D. P. (2016). Application of a new PCR-RFLP panel suggests a restricted population structure for Eimeria tenella in UK and Irish chickens. Veterinary Parasitology, 229, 60-67.

Plattner, F., Yarovinsky, F., Romero, S., Didry, D., Carlier, M. F., Sher, A., & Soldati-Favre, D. (2008). Toxoplasma profilin is essential for host cell invasion and TLR11-dependent induction of an interleukin-12 response. Cell Host & Microbe, 3(2), 77-87.

Reid, A. J., Blake, D. P., Ansari, H. R., Billington, K., Browne, H. P., Bryant, J., & Pain, A. (2014). Genomic analysis of the causative agents of coccidiosis in domestic chickens. Genome Research, 24(10), 1676-1685.

Rose, M. E. (1987). Immunity to Eimeria Infections. Veterinary Immunology and Immunopathology, 17(1-4), 333-343.

Rugarabamu, G., Marq, J. B., Guérin, A., Lebrun, M., & Soldati-Favre, D. (2015). Distinct contribution of T oxoplasma gondii rhomboid proteases 4 and 5 to micronemal protein protease 1 activity during invasion. Molecular Microbiology, 97(2), 244-262.

Shah, M. A. A., Song, X., Xu, L., Yan, R., & Li, X. (2011). Construction of DNA vaccines encoding Eimeria acervulina cSZ-2 with chicken IL-2 and IFN-γ and their efficacy against poultry coccidiosis. Research in Veterinary Science, 90(1), 72-77.

Shirley, M. W., Smith, A. L., & Tomley, F. M. (2005). The biology of avian Eimeria with an emphasis on their control by vaccination. Advances in Parasitology, 60, 285-330.

Smith, N. C., Wallach, M., Petracca, M., Braun, R., & Eckert, J. (1994). Maternal transfer of antibodies induced by infection with Eimeria maxima partially protects chickens against challenge with Eimeria tenella. Parasitology, 109(5), 551-558.

Song, H., Qiu, B., Yan, R., Xu, L., Song, X., & Li, X. (2013). The protective efficacy of chimeric SO7/IL-2 DNA vaccine against coccidiosis in chickens. Research in Veterinary Science, 94(3), 562-567.

Song, X., Gao, Y., Xu, L., Yan, R., & Li, X. (2015). Partial protection against four species of chicken coccidia induced by multivalent subunit vaccine. Veterinary Parasitology, 212(3-4), 80-85.

Song, X., Xu, L., Yan, R., Huang, X., Shah, M. A. A., & Li, X. (2009). The optimal immunization procedure of DNA vaccine pcDNA–TA4–IL-2 of Eimeria tenella and its cross-immunity to Eimeria necatrix and Eimeria acervulina. Veterinary Parasitology, 159(1), 30-36.

Takala, S. L., & Plowe, C. V. (2009). Genetic diversity and malaria vaccine design, testing and efficacy: preventing and overcoming 'vaccine resistant malaria'. Parasite Immunology, 31(9), 560-573.

Vrba, V., & Pakandl, M. (2015). Host specificity of turkey and chicken Eimeria: controlled cross-transmission studies and a phylogenetic view. Veterinary Parasitology, 208(3-4), 118-124.

Wallach, M. G., Ashash, U., Michael, A., & Smith, N. C. (2008). Field application of a subunit vaccine against an enteric protozoan disease. PLoS One, 3(12), e3948.

Wang, Q., Chen, L., Li, J., Zheng, J., Cai, N., Gong, P., & Zhang, X. (2014). A novel recombinant BCG vaccine encoding Eimeria tenella rhomboid and chicken IL-2 induces protective immunity against coccidiosis. The Korean Journal of Parasitology, 52(3), 251.

Williams, R. B. (1999). A compartmentalised model for the estimation of the cost of coccidiosis to the world's chicken production industry. International Journal forParasitology, 29(8), 1209-1229.

Williams, R. B., Marshall, R. N., Pagès, M., Dardi, M., & del Cacho, E. (2009). Pathogenesis of Eimeria praecox in chickens: virulence of field strains compared with laboratory strains of E. praecox and Eimeria acervulina. Avian Pathology, 38(5), 359-366.

Yin, G., Lin, Q., Qiu, J., Qin, M., Tang, X., Suo, X., & Liu, X. (2015). Immunogenicity and protective efficacy of an Eimeria vaccine candidate based on Eimeria tenella immune mapped protein 1 and chicken CD40 ligand. Veterinary Parasitology, 210(1-2), 19-24.

Zhang, L., Liu, R., Ma, L., Wang, Y., Pan, B., Cai, J., & Wang, M. (2012). Eimeria tenella: expression profiling of toll-like receptors and associated cytokines in the cecum of infected day-old and three-week old SPF chickens. Experimental Parasitology, 130(4), 442-448.

12

Phyto-Adsorbents Tool for Amelioration of Mycotoxins in Poultry Feed

[1]Swathi Bora, [2]Gurram Srinivas, [3]Divya Begari, [4]S. Sai Reddy, [5]M. Hanumanth Rao and [6]Sushmasri Kandanulu

[1]*Department of Veterinary Pathology*
[2,4,]*Poultry Research Station*
[3]*NDRI, Karnal*
[5]*Principal, AHP, Mamnoor*
[6]*ICAR -DPR*
P.V. Narsimha Rao Telangana Veterinary University, Rajendranagar Hyderabad, Telangana

Mycotoxins are naturally occurring toxic secondary metabolites produced by molds. More than 25% of world's food crops are contaminated with mycotoxins (Eskola *et al.*, 2020). Like other environmental pollutants, mycotoxins also harm the health and productivity of animals and poultry. Mycotoxin development typically occurs in the field, during feed processing and storage under unfavourable conditions. Factors such as temperature changes, storage time, and conditions play a crucial role in fungal growth and aflatoxin synthesis. India's poultry industry suffers substantial economic losses due to widespread mycotoxin exposure, leading to reduced growth rates, compromised feed conversion efficiency, lower carcass yield, and compromised quality. The heightened vulnerability to diseases is attributed to the immunosuppressive effects on affected birds (Patil *et al.*, 2014).

Herbal extracts have gained prominence as natural and sustainable alternatives for mycotoxin binding in animal and poultry feeds. Designed to neutralize toxins and inhibit fungal toxin production, these extracts effectively manage mycotoxicosis. Specific formulations show positive outcomes, including enhanced weight gain, improved feed efficiency, reduced mortality rates, and increased liveability in poultry (Giannenas *et al.*, 2022). The use of Phyto adsorbents has recently emerged as a promising way to counter mycotoxicosis. The term Phyto adsorbent refers to typically plant-based materials or plants themselves that are employed to remove or immobilize pollutants, such as heavy metals, organic chemicals, and other toxins.

In recent times, herbs such as *Andrographis Paniculata, Boerhavia Diffusa, Emblica Officinalis, Terminalia chebula, Phyllanthus niruri, and Solanum Nigrum* have been utilized individually or in combination as ameliorative agents against mycotoxins. These herbal interventions have demonstrated a positive synergistic impact, mitigated the detrimental effects of mycotoxins and nullified their harmful consequences.

Andrographis paniculata

Andrographis paniculata, or Kalmegh, a member of the Acanthaceae family, is an annual herb native to India and Sri Lanka. Revered as the "King of Bitter," its extracts exhibit significant antimicrobial efficacy against various fungi, including A. flavus and Fusarium spp (Yadav *et al.*, 2006). Additionally, Kalmegh demonstrates anti-inflammatory, antihyperglycemic, oxygen radical scavenging, hepatoprotective, and anti-cancer activities both in vivo and in vitro. Hepatoprotective compounds found in Kalmegh leaves, such as neo-andrographolide and andrographolide, contribute to its antioxidant and anti-inflammatory properties (Thakur *et al.*, 2016).

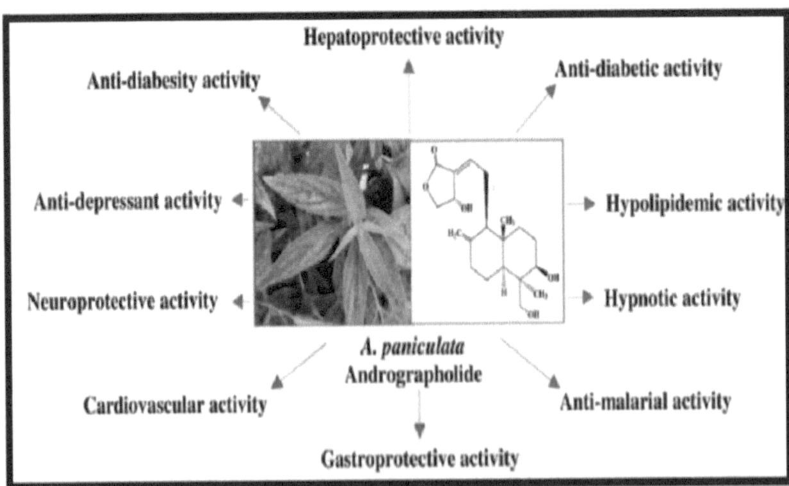

Major phytochemical constituent of *Andrographis paniculate*

Andrographis paniculata aqueous extract at a 300 mg dose exhibited hepatoprotective effects in rats exposed to D-galactosamine (Nasir *et al.*, 2013). In vitro, andrographolide (30 µmol) protected liver cells against CCl4 toxicity (Krithika *et al.*, 2013). Broiler supplementation with Andrographis paniculata in feed increased average daily gain (ADG), reduced feed conversion ratio (FCR), promoted growth, improved live weight, and decreased mortality rate.

Boerhavia diffusa

Boerhavia diffusa, or Punarnava, a plant from the Nyctaginaceae family, is rich in compounds such as flavonoids, alkaloids, steroids, triterpenoids, lipids, carbohydrates, proteins, and glycoproteins (Sahu *et al.*, 2008). Punarnava extract with polyphenols, flavonoids, and tannins exhibits nephroprotective properties (Kalaivani *et al.*, 2015). Punarnavine, an alkaloid in Punarnava, acts as an anticancer, antiestrogenic, antiamoebic, and immunomodulatory agent, enhancing immune system aspects like cellularity and proliferation.

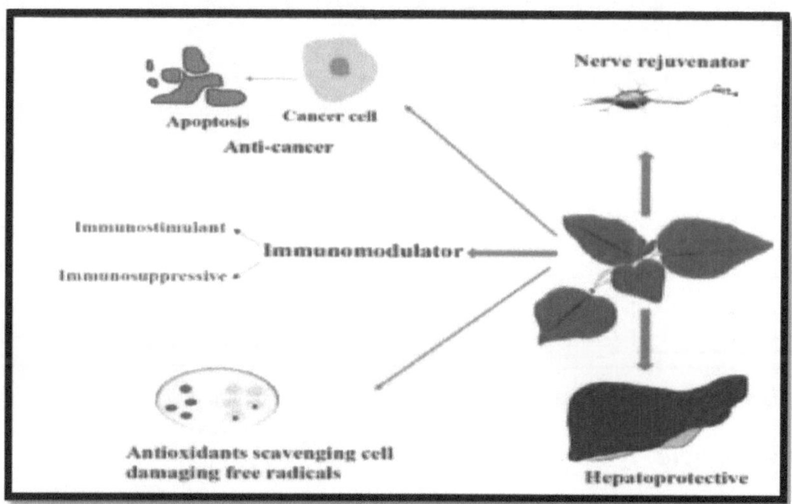

Various pharmacological effects of *Boerhavia diffusa*

Emblica officinalis

Emblica officinalis, commonly known as Indian gooseberry or Amla, is a prominent herb in Indian traditional medicine and a key component of 'Triphala.' Its phytochemical profile includes tannins, alkaloids, phenolic compounds, vitamin C, gallic acid, ellagic acid, chebulinic acid, chebulagic acid, emblicanin-a, emblicanin-b, punigluconin, pedunculagin, citric acid, ellagitannin, trigallayl glucose, pectin, 1-o-galloyl-beta-d-glucose, 3,6-di-o-galloyl-d-glucose, corilagin, 3-ethylgallic acid, isostrictiniin, and flavonoids like quercetin and kaempferol-3-o-alpha-l (6 00 methyl) rhamnopyranoside (Mirunalini and Krishnaveni, 2010).

The aqueous extract of Emblica officinalis demonstrated significant antifungal activity against eight Aspergillus species (*Aspergillus candidus, A. columnaris, A. flavipes, A. flavus, A. fumigatus, A. niger, A. ochraceus, and A. tamari*). Amla supplementation exhibited notable hepato-carcinogenicity inhibition induced by N-nitrosodiethylamine (Chen *et al.*, 2011). Additionally, in broilers, Emblica officinalis supplementation improved body weight significantly (Naik *et al.*, 2020) and demonstrated a protective effect against induced aflatoxicosis (Khetmalis *et al.*, 2018).

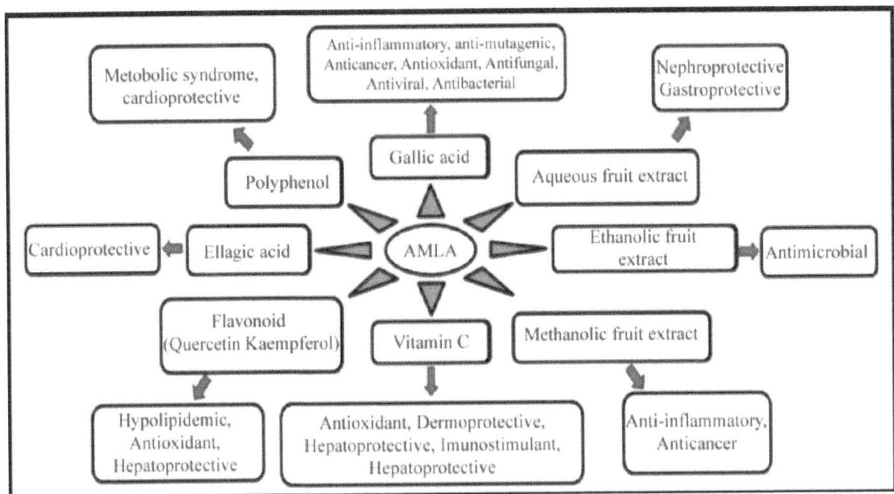

Therapeutic activities of solvent extract and compounds of *Emblica officinalis*

Terminalia chebula

Terminalia chebula, or Haritaki/Myrobalan, a key component of Triphala, has a rich history in traditional medicine, renowned for cathartic effects (Narendra and Manasi, 2021). Its pharmacological activities encompass antioxidant properties from chebulic acid, hepato-protectivity, neuroprotectivity, antidiabetic, and anti-inflammatory effects. Abundant tannins like gallic acid, ellagic acid, chebulic acid (Balakrishna and Lakshmi, 2017), and saccharides are present.

In poultry, *Terminalia chebula* in feed enhances hematological and productivity parameters, demonstrating antimicrobial effects against E. coli and salmonella, common poultry pathogens.

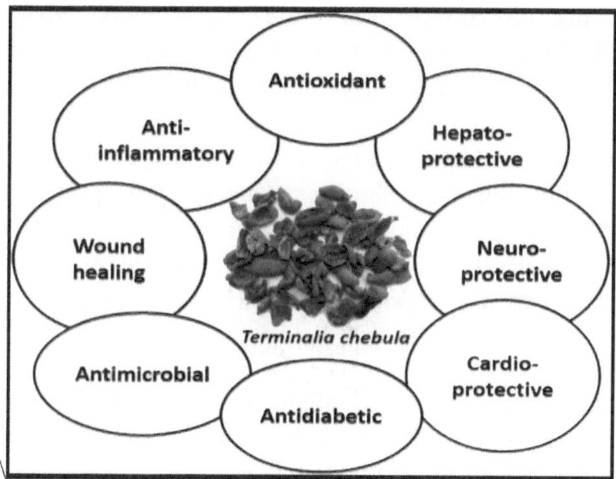

Representation of some pharmacological activities of *Terminalia chebula*

Phyllanthus niruri

Phyllanthus, particularly *Phyllanthus niruri* L. (Bhumi Amlaki), stands out as a extensively studied genus for liver disorders, belonging to the Euphorbiaceae family. This wild herb, easily cultivated in diverse geographies, is rich in bioactive compounds like flavonoids, lignans, tannins, coumarins, terpenes, phenylpropanoids, and saponins. Traditional use of this medicinal herb aligns with its therapeutic properties. Key bioactive compounds identified include hypophyllanthin, catechin, epicatechin, rutin, quercetin, chlorogenic acid, ellagic acid, caffeic acid, malic acid, and gallic acid, known for antibacterial properties. Phytochemicals like protocatechuic acid, niruriflavone, and pectolinarin exhibit hepatoprotective effects.

The effect of *Phyllanthus niruri L* reported that 1% of *P. niruri L.* powder added to chicken rations containing aflatoxins B1 (100 ppb) showed better performance than chickens without the 1% *P. niruri L.* powder (Sundaresan *et al.*, 2007) and also could improve the body weight of broilers (Jagadeeswaran and Selvasubramanian, 2014).

Solanum nigrum

Solanum nigrum Linn. is a commonly used traditional herbal plant for various ailments, and it is well known for its therapeutic properties and traditional Indian medicine. *Solanum nigrum* belongs to the Solanaceae family (Oh *et al.*, 2016), also known by Black nightshade or Makoi (Shivappa *et al.*, 2019). Solanum nigrum contains anthocyanins, flavonoids, tannins, gallic acid, quercetin, vitamins C and E, along with trace elements like iron, zinc, and selenium. These components combat oxidation, preventing oxidative stress, liver toxicity, and metabolic disorders, such as diabetes, cardiovascular diseases, and cancer (Saibu *et al.*, 2020). Elhag *et al.* (2011) demonstrated that water and methanolic extracts of Solanum nigrum exhibited hepatoprotective effects in rats with carbon tetrachloride-induced liver damage, reducing serum enzyme levels and bilirubin concentration. This suggests potential for mitigating liver injury. Supplementation of Solanum nigrum in broilers improved liver function and positively influenced serum lipid profiles in broiler chickens, indicating potential benefits for poultry health (Manan *et al.*, 2012).

Conclusion

The incorporation of phyto-adsorbents into aflatoxin-contaminated diets demonstrated significant ameliorative effects, highlighting their promising role in mitigating the adverse impacts of mycotoxins in broilers. This research provides valuable insights into the potential use of phyto-adsorbents as effective supplements for poultry nutrition to enhance growth performance and alleviate the detrimental effects of mycotoxins.

13

Fetal Programming An Innovative Approach for Management of Heat Stress in Poultry

Vaishali Gupta[1], Amitav Bhattacharyya[2] and Pankaj Kumar Shukla[2]

[1]Gyeongsang National University, Republic of Korea
[2] Deen Dayal Upadhyaya Pashu Chikitsa Vigyan Vishwavidyalaya, DUVASU Mathura, Uttar Pradesh 281 001

The thermal range ideal for poultry rearing is 13°C to 24°C and is known as thermo neutral zone. Any temperature on either side of this zone falls in the critical range (24°C-38°C and 0-13°C) and is detrimental to birds. Heat stress (HS) happens when the amount of heat produced by a bird exceeds the bird's capability to dissipate the heat from the body to its surrounding environment both by sensible and insensible heat loss. The imbalance between heat production and dissipation result due to variations in a combination of various factors *viz.* sunlight, temperature of the air, humidity etc. and individual variations at bird level *viz.* sex, breed, species and physiological status (Lara and Rostagno, 2013). During heat stress, the birds reduce their heat production by decreased feed intake and increased water consumption. Thus, presently HS is a great concern worldwide particularly in the tropical and subtropical areas.

The physiological consequences of HS may be briefly listed as raised core body temperature, decreased feed intake and energy availability to cells, alteration in electrolyte balance and blood pH, digestibility along with metabolism of various nutrients, increased circulatory corticosterone levels and depressed immunity, endocrine and reproductive functions (Yahav, 2009; Syafwan*et al.* 2011 and Renaudeau*et al.*, 2012). Oxidative stress is associated with heat stress as there is an increase in cellular energy demand. Thus, increased mitochondrial energy generation results in overproduction of ROS due to decreased mitochondrial respiratory chain activity (Yang *et al.* , 2010) and high mitochondrial oxygen concentrations (Green *et al.*, 2004). Excess amount of ROS enhances lipid peroxidation, decreases vitamin concentrations, induces mitochondrial dysfunction and stress gene expression leading to dysfunction in antioxidant enzymes and DNA damage. Thus, efforts have been made for the mitigation of heat stress in poultry by various approaches. However, in recent years, novel approaches like nutritional manipulation and thermal conditioning have been tried for mitigation of heat stress in poultry (Daghir, 2008 and Lin *et al.*, 2006).

Nutritional Manipulation

Nutrition plays a pivotal role in alleviating heat stress. Hence, various nutritional strategies have been attempted to ameliorate the adverse effects of heat stress *viz.* decreasing protein level and dietary amino acid composition, increasing the intake of fat and supplementing betaine (Balnave and Brake, 2005; Daghir, 2009; Gous and Morris, 2005; Lin *et al.*, 2006). Increased ambient temperature resulted in decreased micro minerals and vitamins concentrations in serum and increased excretion (Khan *et al.*, 2012). Hence, supplementing potent anti-oxidants like micro nutrients and vitamins may be useful (Yun *et al.*, 2012). Vitamins A, E, C, Zn and Se supplementation in poultry ration during increased environmental temperature considerably influence the antioxidant status of poultry. The aforesaid nutrients aid processes against lipid peroxidation, improve performance and immune status of the birds.

Minimizing total protein intake with a proper balance of amino acids may help in ameliorating the undesirable effects of heat stress. An imbalanced diet results in excess excretion of nitrogenous wastes thereby resulting in accumulation of aerial ammonia (Carlile, 1984; Kristensen and Wathes, 2000; Miles *et al.*, 2004). The ammonia emissions in poultry house may be amplified by raised environmental temperature (Pratt *et al.*, 2004). Increased ammonia levels may adversely influence the broiler chickens' ability to control effectively their body temperature (Yahav, 2004). Hence, it is needed to accentuate the ideal amino acids for chickens during raised ambient temperature and further studies in this area are warranted.

Other feeding strategies include temporary feed restriction and dual feeding program. Provisional feed restriction prior to heat exposure is an effective way to enhance thermal tolerance. Withdrawal of feed leads to less heat production and reduces mortality of broilers (Francis *et al.*, 1991; Yalçin *et al.*, 2001). However, such feeding regimen may hamper growth rate. Dual feeding programme is another strategy to mitigate heat stress in broilers. This includes feeding diet rich in protein during the cooler phase and rich in energy during the warmer phase of the day. It has been observed that dual feeding decreases the body temperature and mortality while exposure of birds to higher temperature (Basilio *et al.*, 2001).

Thermal Conditioning

Early heat conditioning (EHC) holds promise in eliciting the heat tolerance of broiler chickens. EHC refers to exposing broilers to high temperature (36°C) for 24 h at juvenile stage i.e. 3 to 5 days of age. It has been seen that EHC stimulates the capability of heat tolerance in broilers at later stages of growth (Arjona *et al.*, 1988, 1990; Yahav and Hurwitz, 1996; Zhou *et al.*, 1997). It has been further observed that EHC chickens have lesser body temperature at normal or raised environmental temperature (Basilio *et al.*, 2001; 2003) indicating change in the metabolic status of birds.

Recently, fetal programming by nutritional manipulation and thermal conditioning has been attempted for amelioration of heat stress in poultry.

Fetal Programming

Fetal programming, also called developmental programming or fetal developmental programming is a typical reaction to a specific challenge in mammals during a key developmental time window, which quantitatively and/or qualitatively alters the developmental trajectory with long term effects (Nathanielsz *et al.*, 2007). However, unlike placental mammals the route of transferring the maternal effects is the egg. It has already been envisaged that there occurs maternal transfer of antibodies to off springs from the serum of breeder birds through their yolk sac (Bhattacharyya, 2018).

Fetal Programming with Nutritional Manipulation

Nutritional manipulation may be done either by manipulation of the breeder diet or *in ovo* feeding of nutrients.

Breeder Diet Manipulation

Excess or deficiency of nutrients during or after pregnancy may influence the development of offspring. An adequate maternal nutrition elicits placental growth and nutrient transport as well as vascular development (Belkacemi *et al.*, 2010). Further, maternal nutrient supply impacts the programming of the fetal development and may have unrelenting consequences on anatomy and physiology of offsprings (Godfrey and Barker, 2001). However, in case of oviparous avians, the mechanism is entirely different. It has already been established transfer of maternal IgY antibodies from dam's blood into egg yolks by IgY receptors in ovarian follicles occurs in birds (Cutting and Roth, 1973; Loeken and Roth, 1983) and subsequently IgY is transferred via embryonic circulation from egg yolks to offsprings. Thus, the concept may also hold true for maternal transfer of nutrients and fetal imprinting, though it needs to be studied. Modulation of growth and immunity in offsprings by breeder diet manipulation has been studied in turkeys (Bhattacharyya *et al.*, 2014). It was found that chicks hatched from breeders reared on a elevated plane of nutrition were heavier. In another study, it was reported that *in ovo* feeding of amino acids, essential fatty acids and certain vitamins yielded better post hatch growth and breeders maintained on elevated plane of nutrition and thereafter subjected to *in ovo* feeding of amino acids resulted in enhanced post-hatch immunity (Bhattacharyya *et al.* 2018). However, effect of breeder diet on fetal programming against heat stress is yet to be verified.

In ovo Feeding

In recent years, *in ovo* feeding of vital nutrients improved the growth of late term embryos and post-hatch immunity as well as expression of growth and immunity related genes in poultry (Bhanja *et al.*, 2004; Bhanja *et al.*, 2014; Bhanja*et al.*, 2015a; Nayak*et al.*, 2015; Goel *et al.*, 2015, Bhattacharyya *et al.*, 2018). Bhanja *et al.*, (2015b) studied the effect of *in ovo* administration of nano silver (Nano Ag) in combination with amino acids and reported that there was an augmentation of humoral and cell mediated gene expressions in late term embryo challenged with lipopolysaccharide (LPS) at day 19 of incubation in chicken. In another study, Li *et al.* (2016) noted that *in ovo* feeding of folic acid improves hatchability, FCR, IgG and IgM concentrations. Further, folate metabolism is also improved resulting in enhanced immunity of birds. It was found that histone methylation of IL2 and IL4 promoters and inhibition on the IL6 promoter lead to splenic expression up-regulation. The enhanced growth and immune response by *in ovo* feeding in the aforesaid studies may also have been due to epigenetic modifications of the stress controlling systems which need to be studied. Further, studies on *in ovo* feeding for fetal programming to heat stress are also limited.

Supplementation of vitamin A, C and E in poultry feed help to mitigate heat stress as they serve as potential antioxidants. Zn and Se supplementation in poultry feed also influence the antioxidant status of birds during exposure to high temperature. Betaine too has a role in alleviating heat stress. It has already been illustrated that betaine is a methyl donor and betaine undergo various chemical reactions leading to production of methionine (Anderson *et al.*, 2012). Thereafter, methionine is converted to S-adenosyl methionine, which donates methyl groups to DNA methyl transferase. Ratriyanto *et al.* (2009)

noted that methyl donor supplementation in poultry feed resulted in beneficial effects on intestinal cells and gut microflora. However, embryonic imprinting for heat tolerance through the supplementation of different nutrients acting as antioxidants and also methyl donors like betaine is yet to be ascertained.

Fetal programming by Thermal Conditioning

Manipulation of the environment during embryonic development has long lasting effects on the resulting phenotypes including physiological adaptation required for generating heat resistance. Hence, thermal manipulation during incubation may be a plausible tool to modulate performance, health and well-being during later life. Several studies have noted positive effects of thermal manipulation during incubation resulting in improved heat resistance when birds have been thermally challenged (Collin *et al.*, 2011; Druyan *et al.*, 2012). Resistance to high ambient temperature has been accompanied by changes in metabolism and levels of corticosterone and thyroid hormone. Heat conditioning significantly increased levels of corticosterone, PO_2 and blood pH but decreased PCO_2 at day 14 of incubation followed by a significant depression of T4 level on day 15. However, the aforesaid attributes were back to normal at day 16 of incubation as in control embryos. It has been observed that epigenetic thermal conditioning involves changes in these physiological attributes and probably serve as means for epigenetic temperature adaptation as such processes are also engaged for adapting to heat stress during post-embryonic growth (Moraes *et al.*, 2004). However, molecular mechanisms involving such epigenetic adaptations have to be deduced.

Conclusion

Nutritional manipulation and early age thermal conditioning plays a key role in mitigating heat stress. However, fetal programming involving nutritional and thermal treatments in poultry is still at its infancy unlike mammals. Though, recently studies have been initiated on this aspect but epigenetic modifications with manipulation of the breeder diet and *in ovo* feeding of nutrients and antioxidants have to be studied. Further, studies are also warranted in molecular mechanisms behind epigenetic adaptations involving prenatal thermal conditioning.

References

Anderson OS, Sant KE and Dolinoy DC. Nutrition and epigenetics:an interplay of dietary methyl donors, one-carbon DNA methylation. J NutrBiochem. 2012;23: 853–859.

Arjona AA, Denbow DM and Weaver WD. Effect of heat stress early in life on mortality of broilers exposed to high temperature just prior to marketing. Poult Sci. 1988;67: 226-231.

Arjona AA, Denbow DM and Weaver WD. Neonatal induced thermotolerance: physiological responses. Comp Biochem Physiol. 1990;A95: 393-399.

Balnave D and Brake J. Nutrition and management of heat-stressed pullets and laying hens. World's PoultSci J. 2005;61(3): 399–406.

Basilio, V DE, Requena, F, Leon, A, Vilarino, M and Picard M. Early age thermal conditioning immediately reduces body temperature of broiler chicks in a tropical environment. Poult Sci.2003;82:1235-1241.

Basilio V DE, Vilarino, M, Yahav S and Picard M.Early age thermal conditioning and a dual feeding program for male broilers challenged by heat stress.Poult Sci.2001;80: 29-36.

Belkacemi L, Nelson DM, Desai M, Ross MG. Maternal under nutrition influences placental-fetal development. Biol. Reprod. 2010;83:325–331.

Bhanja, SK, Goel A, Pandey N, Mehra M, Majumdar S and Mandal AB. In ovo carbohydrate supplementation modulates growth and immunity-related genes in broiler chickens. J. Anim. Physiol. Anim. Nutr. 2015a;99:163-173.

Bhanja SK, Mandal AB and Goswami TK. Effect of in ovo injection of amino acids on growth, immune response, development of digestive organs and carcass yields of broiler.Indian J. Poult. Sci. 2004;39:212-218.

Bhanja SK, Sudhagar M, Goel A, Pandey N, Mehra M, Agarwal SK and Mandal AB. Differential expression of growth and immunity related genes influenced by in ovo supplementation of amino acids in broiler chickens. Czech J. Anim. Sci. 2014;59: 399-408.

Bhattacharyya A, Majumdar S, Bhanja SK, Mandal AB, Dash BB and Kadam MM. Effect of dietary manipulation on production, reproduction and immuno competence traits in turkey breeder hens. Indian J. Anim. Sci. 2014;84 (10): 1113–1116.

Bhattacharyya A, Majumdar S, Bhanja SK, Mandal AB and Kadam M. Effect of maternal dietary manipulation and in ovo injection of nutrients on the hatchability indices, post-hatch growth, feed consumption, feed conversion ratio and immunocompetence traits of turkey poults, J. Applied Anim. Res. 2018;46: 287-294.

Carlile, F.S. Ammonia in poultry houses: A literature review. World's PoultSci J.1984;40: 99-113.

Collin A, Bedrani L, Loyau, T, Mignon-Grasteau, S, MetayerCoustard S, Praud C, De Basillo, V, RequenaRodon F., Bastianelli D, Duclos MJ, Tesseraud S, Berri C and Yahav S. Embryo acclimation; an innovative technique to limit mortality due to thermal stress in chicken. Inra. Prod. Anim. 2011;24:191-198.

Cutting JA and Roth TF.Changes in specific sequestration of protein during transport into the developing oocyte of the chicken.BiochimicaetBiophysicaActa. 1973;298: 951–955.

Daghir, N. J. Nutritional strategies to reduce heat stress in broilers and broiler breeders. Lohmann Information.2009;44(1): 6–15.

Druyan S, Piestun, Y and Yahav S. Heat stress in domestic fowl: genetic and physiological aspects. Pages 1-30 in Heat Stress-Causes, Treatment and Prevention, S. Josipovic, and E. Ludwig, eds. Nova Science Publications Inc.2012;New York, NY.

Francis CA, Macleod MG and Anderson JEM. Alleviation of acute heat stress by feed withdrawal or darkness. British Poult Sci. 1991;32: 219-225.

Godfrey KM and Barker DJ.Fetal programming and adult health.Public Health Nutr.2001; 4: 611–624.

Goel A, Bhanja SK, Mehra M, Mandal AB and PandeV.. In ovo trace element supplementation enhances expression of growth genes in embryo and immune genes in post-hatch broiler chickens. J SciFood Agri.doi: 10.1002/jsfa.7438. Epub 2015 Sep 24.

Gous RM and Morris TR. Nutritional interventions in alleviating the effects of high temperatures in broiler production. Proceedings of the Nutrition Society.2005;61(3): 463–475.

Green K, Brand MD, Murphey MP. Prevention of mitochondrial oxidative damage as a therapeutic strategy in diabetes.Diabetes. 2004;53:S110–8

Khan R, Naz S, Nikousefat Z, Selvaggi M, Laudadio V and Tufarelli V. Effect of ascorbic acid in heat-stressed poultry. World's PoultSci J.2012;68(3):477–490.

Kristensen, HH and Wathes, CM. Ammonia and poultry welfare: a review. World's PoultSci J.2000;56: 235-245.

Lara LJ and Rostagno MH.Impact of heat stress on poultry production. Anim. 2013;3:356–369

Lin H, Jiao HC, Buyse J and Decuypere E. Strategies for preventing heat stress in poultry. World's PoultSci J. 2006;62(1): 71–86.

Loeken MR and Roth TF.Analysis of maternal IgG subpopulations which are transported into the chicken oocyte.Immunology.1983; 49: 21–28.

Miles DM, Branton SL and Lott BD. Atmospheric ammonia is detrimental to the performance of modern commercial broilers. Poult Sci. 2004;83: 1650-1654.

Moraes V, Bruggeman V, Malheiros RD and Collin A.The effect of timing of thermal conditioning during incubation on embryo physiological parameters and its relationship to thermotolerance in adult broiler chickens.J. Thermal Biol. 2004;29(1):55-61.

Nathanielsz PW, Poston L and Taylor PD. In utero exposure to maternal obesity and diabetes: Animal models that identify and characterize implications for future health. Clinics in Perinatol.2007;34 (4):515-526.

Nayak N, Rajini RA, Ezhilvalavan S, Kirubaharan J, Sahu AR and Manimaran K. Effect of in ovo feeding of arginine and/or tryptophan on hatchability and small intestinal morphology in broiler chicken. Indian J Poult Sci.2015;50:18-23.

Pratt EV, Rose SP and Keeling AA.Effect of moisture content and ambient temperature on the gaseous nitrogen loss from stores laying hen manure. British Poult Sci.2004;45:301-305.

Ratriyanto A, Mosenthin R, Bauer E and Eklund M. Metabolic, osmoregulatory and nutritional functions of betaine in monogastric animals. Asian-Australasian J Anim Sci. 2009;22:1461-1476.

Renaudeau D, Collin A, Yahav S, De Basilio V, Gourdine JL and Collier RJ. Adaptation to hot climate and strategies to alleviate heat stress in livestock production. Anim. 2012;6:707–728

Syafwan S, Kwakkel RP and Verstegen MWA.Heat stress and feeding strategies in meat-type chickens. World's PoultSci J. 2011;67:653–673.

Yahav S. Alleviating heat stress in domestic fowl: different strategies. World's PoultSci J. 2009;65:719–32.

Yahav S. Ammonia affects performance and thermoregulation of male broiler chickens. Anim Res 2004;53: 289-293.

Yahav S and Hurwitz S. Induction of thermotolerance in male broiler chickens by temperature conditioning at an early age.Poult Sci. 1996;75: 402-406.

Yalçin S, Özkan S, Türkmut L and Siegel PB. Responses to heat stress in commercial and local broiler stocks. 1. Performance traits. British Poult Sci. 2001;42: 149-152.

Yang L, Tan GY, Fu YQ, Feng JH and Zhang M H..Effects of acute heat stress and subsequent stress removal on function of hepatic mitochondrial respiration, ROS production and lipid peroxidation in broiler chickens. Comp Biochem Physiology Part C: Toxicol and Pharmacol. 2010;151(2): 204–208.

Yun SH, Moon YS, Sohn SH and Jang IS. Effects of cyclic heat stress or Vitamin C supplementation during cyclic heat stress on HSP70, inflammatory cytokines, and the antioxidant defense system in Sprague Dawley rats. Exp. Anim.2012;61(5):543–553.

Zhou WT, Fujita M, Ito T and Yamamoto S. Effects of early heat exposure on thermoregulatory responses and blood viscosity of broilers prior to marketing. Br Poult Sci.1997;38:301-306.

14

Fly Control in Poultry Production Best Management Practice

M.A. Gole, D.N. Desai, A.S. Ranade and S.S. Gaikwad

Department of Poultry Science, Mumbai Veterinary College, Parel, Maharashtra Animal and Fishery Science University, Nagpur, Maharashtra

Poultry holds significant value as it provides essential protein, vitamins, and mineral nutrients, including eggs and chicken meat.Poultry is a significant source of organic fertilizer and generates income and employment for millions of farmers and other poultry cultivators. The bigger and richer the industry, the more problems they face.Infectious diseases transmitted by flies, majorly house flies *(Musca domestica*) and other insects are the primary concern for poultry farmers on their farm. The threat of flies is a major problem worldwide wherever poultry farming is an important economic activity.In livestock and medical treatments, flies are significant pests that can cause irritation, spoilage of food, and serve as vectors for various pathogenic organisms. They are also highly destructive.

Food security is a major issue today, and the theme of this World Health Day is "Food Security from Farm to Fork. One of the main reasons for these food safety concerns is the problem of flies in farms, which not only reduces production but also causes food safety problems for humans. The illegal use of antibiotics and chemicals to solve these problems also increases the threat to food safety as these harmful chemicals directly affect birds. The growing fly population poses a threat to the health of people around farms, the deterioration of community relations and the risk of disease outbreaks. The transmission of diseases from flies to humans and animals involves more than 100 organisms, such as protozoa, bacteria, viruses, rickettsia, molds, or worms.

Flies are attracted to chickens due to the presence of chicken manure, wet food, dirt, and bedding. The moisture and ammonia in the manure, as well as the feed and growth of the farm, help create a favorable environment for flies to attack.The establishment of physical barriers and the appropriate spraying of pesticides is among the methods used by farmers. Although these methods are effective by themselves, they are time-consuming and expensive for the farmer, but the pesticides that are available in the market affect the food of the animals.

Flies are considered intermediate hosts for the worms and can transmit roundworms to birds in captivity. Flies carry mites and other nematode products on their feet, from dung to dung, food, and water.For humans and poultry alike, flies pose a great health risk. They are potential intermediate hosts of *Salmonella, Campylobacter* and *E. Coli* which have a deteriorating health effect on poultry.The speed at which flies reproduce varies depending on environmental factors such as temperature, humidity and food sources, but five or six generations are not uncommon in a single breeding season.Infected flies are eaten by bird feeders. Chemical products such as organophosphates, organochlorines, pyrethrins, etc. When farmers use it to control the fly menace on their farms, it provides a temporary solution, but farmers don't know what the cost will be. These chemicals cause the flies to develop resistance to these chemicals, so higher doses must be used or the insecticides used must be replaced regularly to prevent the development of resistance. The side effects of poultry products with these chemicals increase, especially at higher doses. In recent years, the prevention and residue of dangerous substances in food are already being reported, and until now the control measures to check these food safety problems are the worst.

Ammonia Production and Fly Hazard

The production of ammonia in poultry farms is due to the breakdown of nitrogen-containing compounds in the poultry waste, and when this production ends, the amount of ammonia produced is also greater, and certainly more ammonia is produced as a result of poor protein metabolism or poor liver function. Poor protein metabolism causes many adverse effects on the bird's health, and therefore requires rapid treatment to control the correct functioning of the liver. Flies are attracted to the smell of ammonia, nitrogen and amino-containing compounds produced on the farm, and the flies can smell it from a distance.

Life Cycle of Flies

Flies complete their life cycle in a unique sequence of life stages: egg, larva, pupa, and adult.The life cycle of a fly can vary between week to one month. In rotting, decaying, or fermenting organic stuff (such as waste, manure, etc.) with a moisture content of between 50 and 85%, flies breed and lay their eggs.

Poultry litter is particularly favorable as a medium for the development of fly populations because it contains a moisture level of about 75%-80%.The life cycle of the fly varies with temperature, about 10 days at 85°F(29° C), 21 days at 70°F(21°C), and 45 days at 60°F (15.5°C) (West *et al.*, 1951 and Axtell*et al.*, 1986). Temperatures below 50-53°F (10-11.5°C) will not produce flies. In areas with cold winters, mosquitoes hibernate during the period when they may or may not survive as adults outside. No hibernation (development stopped). However, mosquitoes spend the winter indoors, reducing their reproductive activity if they have a suitable environment. Exact values vary, but adult fly activity may begin at an average temperature of 44°F (6.7°C), but flies are still active or crawling at 45–48°F (7.2–8, 9 °C) and 53°F (11.6 °C). Generally, the threshold for outdoor fly activity is 50°F or less (West *et al.*, 1951 and Keiding 1976). Adult flies tend to seek temperatures above 60°F (15.6°C) whenever possible. However, the lower the temperature, the longer rate of survival.

Fly Control Methods

There are four major types of fly control methods:

- Cultural control
- Mechanical control
- Chemical control
- Biological control

1) Cultural Control

Culture methods are the basis of anycontrol program. Biosecurity, waste management; equipment maintenance and resident maintenance (especially humidity and airflow control) are all part of this. These methods are purely based on the management of the farm. To ensure proper air flow and humidity, housing management involves grading and construction to divert rainwater from the house, as well as the appropriate adjustment and operation of fans, vents, and side curtains manure and litter control.The key to litter management is moisture management, cleaning and manure removal. Moist poultry manure is very attractive to adult flies and provides excellent conditions for fly breeding and development. Therefore, manure moisture is the most important factor in flow control. Fresh poultry manure has a moisture content of 75-80%, and flies breed in manure with a moisture content of 50-85% (Neyeloff 1981). Keeping manure or litter as dry as possible is essential for controlling pest populations, especially flies. Keeping vegetation low around homes is essential to ensure proper airflow and to keep rodents out.

- Keep litter dry: Flies lay their eggs in wet manure, so reducing the moisture content to about 30 percent will make it less attractive. Proper ventilation is important to keep the manure dry.
- Regular raking: Removing wet litter and regular raking prevents flies from breeding and interrupting their life cycle. For this, you need enough space for spreading or suitable rooms for storage and composting of manure.
- Avoid water leaks: Repair any leaks in the water system to prevent excess moisture from entering the manure. Also, prevent rain water from entering the manure.
- Use of manure belt: If your farm has a manure belt system, remove manure from the belts two or three times a week. Fresh manure attracts flies, and if not removed quickly enough, flies can thrive. These flies can then continue to develop in manure storage.
- Salt content of feed: Avoid high salt content of feed and treat flock against loose feces.
- Maintain sanitation: daily removal of dead birds and their proper disposal. Minimize spilled bait and broken eggs, as these attract flies. Keep grass and weeds trimmed around sheds to eliminate breeding space for adult flies and improve airflow.

2) Mechanical Control

Mechanical control is the use of tools and devices to control flies.This may involve the use of physical barriers like screens, manure removal devices, and fly traps, electronic repellents, or "bug eliminators" to prevent access to food processing areas. Electric traps are not suitable for handling high flows due to the number of equipment required and their cost, but they can be used in some small areas near product management, offices and areas of interest. A distance of 2 m (or about 6 ft) from the egg handling area is sufficient to prevent houseflies from being bitten by the trap (Pickens 1989).

Manure is typically removed from high rise galleries by small front loaders or skid steer loaders, treated and spread immediately on agricultural fields. New automatic manure removal belt systems and manure drying systems can improve control and reduce flies. Moisture can be reduced when hot air is supplied to the manure belt to dry out the litter. A belt will carry the manure to the end of the row of cages and remove it from the house. High rise composting is another option for manure management as indoor composting machines are available. This approach is a combination of machine control and cultural control, which will be discussed in the next section on cultural control.

3) Chemical Control

Chemical treatments are often required to maintain fly populations in poultry sheds. Farmers should monitor fly populations periodically to evaluate fly control programs and determine when insecticide applications are needed. Keep accurate records of chemicals used and doses. The untimely and inappropriate use of harmful pesticides, along with poor litter management, poor moisture management and sanitation practices, will increase pest populations and the need for additional pesticide applications. However, only approved (registered) insecticides should be used and then in a manner aimed at protecting biological control agents. Unfortunately, insecticides effective against flies are generally toxic to predators and parasites (Axtell 1966, 1968, Axtell and Edwards 1970).

Depending on the type, composition and concentration of the chemical used and the type of surface sprayed, treated areas may remain toxic for 2 to 15 weeks. Applying in areas where flies rest (mainly upper areas where vomit and feces are found) is most effective. These spraysperform poorly on brick or concrete floors in areas exposed to direct sunlight. If flocks are present, a residual spray after manure removal can be effective in reducing fly production that occurs after barn cleaning. The second application should be done 5-6 weeks later.

Residual Sprays: Houses should be thoroughly cleaned and disinfected before insecticides are applied.Protective clothing should be worn while applying insecticide.Mix the insecticide concentrate with clean water according to the manufacturer's recommendations and only use clean sprayers to apply the insecticide.Apply it to non-absorbent house surfaces such as hard wood, painted or coated walls.Allow the insecticide to dry for 2-3 hours.After drying, these products are harmless to poultry and humans.Insecticides remain effective for 2-3 months.

Non – Residual Sprays: Only effective at the time of application and have no long-term effectiveness.It is best used in areas where primary elimination of large fly populations is required. In this case, a no-residue pesticide should be used before applying a long-acting residual pesticide. As with pesticide residues, this application is only suitable for non-toxic home remedies. You can use a fog machine to spray residual pesticides throughout your home.

There are four types of chemical control methods for flies:

a) **Insect Growth Regulators (IGR's) (Cyromazine):** It is added to feed to prevent fly larvae from entering the manure.The IGR process is highly selective and ensures the conservation of natural stream predator populations. IGR can be used for 4 to 6 weeks when new flocks are introduced in the layer or breeder cages. If the fly population continues to increase, treatments can be done every 4 to 6 months. However, it is important not to rely too much on this product. This is because incidences of resistance can arise.

b) **Larvicidal Sprays:** These sprays are directly applied to the manure surface to kill fly larvae.

Group/class	Activeingredients
Herbal	Herbal
Benzoylurea	Diflubenzuron
Carbamate	Thiodicarb
Triazine	Cyromazine
Ether	Pyriproxyfen

c) **Adulticide Sprays:** Theyare used to control adult flies, from both inside and outside the poultry sheds. It can be used as a residual spray or a quick spray. They are to be used sparingly and as a last resort to avoid resistance.

Group/class	Activeingredients
Pyrethroid	Deltamethrin
	Bifenthrin
	Cypermethrin
	Beta-cyfluthrin
	LambdaCyhalothrin
	Alphamethrin
Organophosphate	Chlorpyriphos
	Dichlorovos
Neonicotinoid	Imidacloprid
	Thiamethoxam
Herbal	Herbal

d) **Fly Baits:** Insecticide baits can be utilized to trap and control adult flies for field treatment. Keep them where flies congregate but avoid manure pits to avoid killing the beneficial parasites and predators. Fly paints, like instant paint, attract and kill flies on contact. Apply in clean areas infested with flies.

Group/class	Activeingredients
Herbal	Herbal
Carbamate	Propoxur
Neonicotinoid	Acetamiprid
	Imidacloprid

4) Biological Control

The use of biological pest control is particularly advanced in poultry production to control houseflies and fleas, in which for long-term manure accumulation is carried, especially in cage system rearing of birds (Axtell 1986, 1990, Legner 1995, Wilhoit *et al.* 1991a). There are two main approaches to biological control. This is done by increasing the population of natural enemies with regular releases (Rutz and Patterson 1990). The parasites that kill housefly larvae are sold and released, although they have a varying degree of success. Parasite populations are often present, and the populations can be encouraged to increase by keeping the manure dry enough to allow easy access to the fly's habitat. Also, keeping manure dry can increase the population of fly feeders.

The most common fly predators that inhibit fly populations on poultry farms are *Muscidifuraxraptor Geralt* and *Sanders, M. zaraptor Kogan* and *Legner, Spalangiacameroni Perkins*, and *S. Nigroaenea Curtis* (Geden 1996, Mann *et al.* 1990a, b, Rueda and Axtell 1985, Wilhoit *et al.* 1991c). As a result, keeping manure as dry as possible can encourage the development of different types of manure fauna, which feed on the fly eggs and larvae, thereby reducing fly populations. Promotion of biological control agents through manure management is important in fly control programs in poultry systems involving manure accumulation.

In addition to parasites and predators, a number of pathogens that affect flies occur in poultry production systems aresome strains of the entomopathogenic fungi *Entomophthora muscae* and *Beauveria bassiana* (Balsam) are widespread and suppress fly populations. However, these have not been exploited commercially for fly control.

Conclusion

Fly populations are important to monitor in the poultry houses and their surroundings. It is vital to systematically assess the manure quality and populations of biological control agents and flies. Regular inspection of manure, water sources and water systems is the basis of corrective actions to correct moisture problems. Testing for fly larvae levels can help treat areas where manure is a problem. Monitoring adults using baited traps or location cards is a simple guide to the fly population so you can adjust your fly management practices as needed. Adequate monitoring is required for a fly control program when low-dose pesticides are used.

References

Axtell, R.C., Fly control in confined livestock and poultry production. 1986, Greensboro, NC: CIBA-GEIGY Corporation Tech. Monongraph. 59 p.

Axtell, R.C., Poultry integrated pest management: Status and future. Integrated Pest Mgmt. Rev., 1999. 4: p. 53-73.

Axtell, R.C. Livestock integrated pest management (IPM): Principals and prospects. In Systems Approach to Animal Health and Production: A Symposium, March 31-April 2. 1981. Lexington, KY: University of Kentucky.

Axtell, R.C. Use of predators and parasites in filth fly IPM programs in poultry housing. In Status of Biological Control of Filth Flies, Proc Workshop February 4-5. 1981. Gainesville, FL: USDA.

Geden, C.J. (1996) Modeling host attacks and progeny production of Spalangiagemina, Spalangiacameroni, and Muscidfurax raptor (Hymenoptera: Pteromalidae) at constant and variable temperatures. Biological Control 7, 172–8.

Keiding, J., The housefly - biology and control. 1976, Rept. Wld. Hlth. Org. . p. 89.

Legner, E.F. (1995) Biological control of Diptera of medical and veterinary importance. Journal of Vector Ecology 20, 59–120.

Mann, J.A., Axtell, R.C. and Stinner, R.E. (1990b) Temperature- dependent development and parasitism rates of four species of Pteromalidae (Hymenoptera) parasitoids of house fly (Musca domestica) pupae. Medical and Veterinary Entomology 4, 245–53.

Mann, J.A., Stinner, R.E. and Axtell, R.C. (1990a) Parasitism of house fly (Musca domestica) pupae by four species of Ptero- malidae (Hymenoptera): Effects of host-parasitoid densities and host distribution. Medical and Veterinary Entomology 4, 235–43.

Neyeloff, S., Cultural methods of fly and odor control for poultry farms. Cooperative Extension System, University of Connecticut, 1981. Bulletin 81-40.

Pickens, L.G., *et al.*, Dispersal patterns and populations of the house fly affected by sanitation and weather in rural Maryland. J. Econ. Entomol., 1967. 60: p. 1250-1255.

Pickens, L.G., Factors affecting the distance of scatter of house flies (Diptera: Muscidae) from electronic traps. J. Econ. Entomol., 1989. 82(1): p. 149-151.

Rueda, L.M. and Axtell, R.C. (1985) Guide to common species of pupal parasites (Hymenoptera: Pteromalidae) of the house fly and other muscoid flies associated with poultry and livestock manure. North Carolina Agricultural Research Service Bulletin 278, 1–88.

Rueda, L.M. and Axtell, R.C. (1996) Temperature-dependent development and survival of the lesser mealworm, Alphitobiusdiaperinus (Coleoptera: Tenebrionidae). Medical and Veteri- nary Entomology 10, 80–6.

Rueda, L.M. and Axtell, R.C. (1997) Arthropods in litter of poultry (broiler chicken and turkey) houses. Journal of Agricultural Entomology 14, 81–91.

Stafford, K.C., III and C.H. Collison, Manure pit temperatures and relative humidity of Pennsylvania high-rise poultry houses and their relationship to arthropod population development. Poultry Sci., 1987. 66: p. 1603-1611.

Stafford, K.C., III and D.E. Bay, Dispersion pattern and association of house fly, Musca domestica (Diptera: Muscidae), larvae and both sexes of Macrochelesmuscaedomesticae (Acari: Macrochelidae) in response to poultry manure moisture, temperature, and accumulation. Environ. Entomol, 1986. 16: p. 159-164.

Stafford, K.C., III and D.E. Bay, Dispersion statistics and sample size estimates for house fly (Diptera: Muscidae) larvae and Macrochelesmuscaedomesticae (Acari: Macrochelidae) in poultry manure. J. Med. Entomol., 1994. 31(5): p. 732-737.

Stafford, K.C. and C.H. Collison, Poultry Pest Management for Pennsylvania and the Northeast. Special Circular 338. 1987: The Pennsylvania State University. 10.

Webster, A.B., N. Hinkle, and S.A. Thompson, Commercial egg tip: Can in-house composting reduce flies in high-rise layer houses?, in University of Georgia CES Poutry Tips. 2005.

West, L.S., The house fly: its natural history, medical importance, and control. 1951, Ithaca, NY: Comstock Publ. Co. 584.

Wilhoit, L.R., Axtell, R.C. and Stinner, R.E. (1991b) Estimating manure temperatures from air temperatures and results of its use in models of filth fly (Diptera: Muscidae) development. Environmental Entomology 20, 635–43.

Wilhoit, L.R., Stinner, R.E., Axtell, R.C., Bacheler, J.E. and Mann, J.A. (1991c) PARMOD: A model for Muscidfurax spp. and Spalangia spp. (Hymenoptera: Pteromalidae), parasites of house fly pupae (Diptera: Muscidae). Environmental Entomol- ogy 20, 1418–26.

Wilhoit, L.R., Stinner, R.E. and Axtell, R.C. (1991a) Computer simulation model of house fly management in confined-animal production systems. North Carolina Agricultural Research Service Technical Bulletin 296, 1–81.

Wilhoit, L.R., Stinner, R.E. and Axtell, R.C. (1991d) CARMOD: A simulation model for Carcinopspumilio (Coleoptera: His-teridae) population dynamics and predation on immature stages of house flies (Diptera: Muscidae). Environmental Entomology 20, 1079–88.

15

Combat Wet Litter Issues for A Successful and Profitable Flock

Sushil Prasad[1], Manish K. Singh[2], S.K. Joshi[3] and Anand Prakash[4]

[1]College of Veterinary Science and Animal Husbandry, Ranchi, Birsa Agricultural University, Ranchi, India
[2]Department of Poultry Science, College of Veterinary Science and Animal Husbandry, DUVASU, Mathura, Uttar Pradesh, India
[3]College of Veterinary Science and Animal Husbandry, Orissa University Agricultural Technology, Bhubaneswar, Odisha, India
[4]College of Veterinary Sciences, Guru Angad Dev Veterinary and Animal Sciences University, Rampura Phul, Bathinda Punjab, India

Wet litter can be caused by extrinsic or intrinsic factors related to excessive excretion of water. When the moisture content of litter exceeds 35%, it can lead to various issues, including pododermatitis of the foot pads, resulting in poor growth rate in broilers and low fertility in breeder flocks. Wet litter can also contribute to inflammation of the feather follicles. This can lead to gangrenous dermatitis, which is responsible for downgrading at processing or rejection by consumers. Additionally, wet litter is often associated with outbreaks of coccidiosis, as the oocysts of Eimeria spp. require moisture levels over 25% to mature. Necrotic enteritis occurs frequently in houses with areas of wet litter, while damp litter may contribute to the proliferation of toxic fungi. The bacterial flora of damp litter favors the production of ammonia, which can lead to erosion of the cornea of the eye and respiratory stress if levels exceed a certain threshold.

Causes of Wet Litter

Extrinsic Factors

- "When it's raining, make sure to close all ventilation openings using either shutters or watertight curtains to prevent water from getting inside." **Houses located in areas subject to seasonal monsoon rains should be designed to withstand excessive wind and rain.**
- **Excessive condensation on the underside of the roof:** Under cold ambient temperatures, uninsulated houses develop condensation on the underside of the roof sheeting, which drips onto the litter. Proper ventilation and roof insulation are necessary to fix this issue.
- It's imperative to take action against the problem of leakage from suspended bell drinkers and nipple systems, and the best way to do so is by investigating the root cause and taking appropriate corrective measures. By doing this, you can ensure that your system is functioning at its optimal level, saving you both time and money in the long run. Don't let leaks go unnoticed - act today to prevent any further damage. This may involve the installation of a pressure regulator or filters to prevent particulate matter that clogs valves from entering water lines.

Intrinsic Factors

Excretion of water may occur in the form of urine, known as diuresis, or from the digestive tract. It is important to determine whether the excessive release of fluid from the cloaca, also known as wet droppings, is from the urinary or the digestive tract.

Diarrhoea

The causes of this may include

- **Coccidiosis:** This infection can be diagnosed by examining the intestines of birds that have been sacrificed and have ruffled plumage and paler appearance. The diagnosis is confirmed by examining mucosal scrapings under a microscope. Appropriate therapy (such as sulpha drugs or amprolium) can restore normal function.
- **Bacterial Infections:** These can result in enteritis. Microscopic and microbiological examination of intestines from affected sacrificed birds is required to establish the diagnosis. Appropriate antibiotics, such as tetracycline, neomycin, zinc bacitracin, or ampicillin, should be administered by statutory regulations.
- **Viral Infections:** These can include reovirus and other enteric viral agents that may result in diarrhea, especially in young flocks. Diagnosis

involves electron microscopy of mucosal scrapings and feces, histological examination of intestinal tissue, and viral isolation attempts. Duration is typically a few days to a week. These procedures require a specialized laboratory. There are no specific treatments for viral infections other than supportive therapy, which involves electrolyte supplements and raising the brooding temperature.

- Complex carbohydrates found in wheat, barley, and cassava may not be properly digested in the anterior intestinal tract, leading to digestive problems, bacterial degradation, and diarrhea. It is advisable to replace these cereals with maize and vegetable proteins with high-quality soybean meal. Enzyme combinations that can be obtained commercially can also be used to improve the digestibility of unconventional carbohydrate sources.
- Diarrhea can be caused by mycotoxins such as aflatoxin and fusariotoxins. To determine the presence of these toxins, a feed analysis is necessary. If these toxins are present, it is recommended to substitute the contaminated ingredients or supplement the diet with an effective mycotoxin binder.
- Rancid fat in feed, which may occur due to prolonged storage at high temperatures, can cause diarrhea. Wet droppings, pasty vents, encephalomalacia, immunosuppression, and low growth rates are some of the other negative effects of incorporating non-stabilized fat, byproduct meal, or rice bran into feed.

Diuresis

Birds tend to excrete excessive amounts of water when exposed to high temperatures. This is a natural response to increased water consumption, which helps them to release heat through evaporative cooling via their respiratory system. Drinking cold water can also help birds lower their body temperature by acting as a heat sink in their digestive tract. If a bird's diet contains too much salt, sodium, or chloride, it can result in excessive water intake and diuresis. This may occur due to incorrect formulation, mixing, or accidental contamination of their food. High levels of salt can also be present in fishmeal or carcass meal batches. If birds display symptoms of diuresis or wet droppings after a change in diet or purchasing feed from a new supplier, appropriate analysis should be conducted to determine the cause. Magnesium contamination in limestone used in layer and breeder diets can also lead to diuresis. Water that contains chemical and mineral impurities such as sodium and magnesium can also result in diuresis. This is usually a chronic problem in flocks and can be confirmed through water analysis. Mycotoxins, including ochratoxins, can damage the kidney and lead to excessive water excretion. The presence of this condition can be determined by identifying the specific mycotoxin in feed and examining the kidneys of affected birds under a microscope. Several nephropathogenic viruses can also cause diuresis in flocks during the acute and recovery phases of infection. Acute infectious bursal disease, avian nephrosis virus, and nephropathogenic strains of infectious bronchitis virus are some of these viruses. Skip-a-day feeding of replacement broiler breeder pullets can lead to diuresis due to excessive water intake on non-feed days. Mature hens subject to post-peak restriction often demonstrate excessive water intake and wet droppings. It may be necessary to implement a water restriction program as recommended by the breeder to regulate feed and water intake. However, if the flock is exposed to an ambient temperature above 30°C, it is not advisable to implement such a program.

Effect of Wet Litter on Bird

- **Increase Ammonia levels:** Ammonia produced by the breakdown of uric acid by bacteria in the litter. Did you know that levels greater than 20 ppm have a profound negative effect on poultry performance? It's true! To ensure that your poultry is performing at its best, it's important to keep the levels below this threshold. By doing so, you can guarantee that your poultry will be healthy, happy, and productive. So don't take any chances - make sure to monitor the levels and keep them in check!

- Respiratory problems

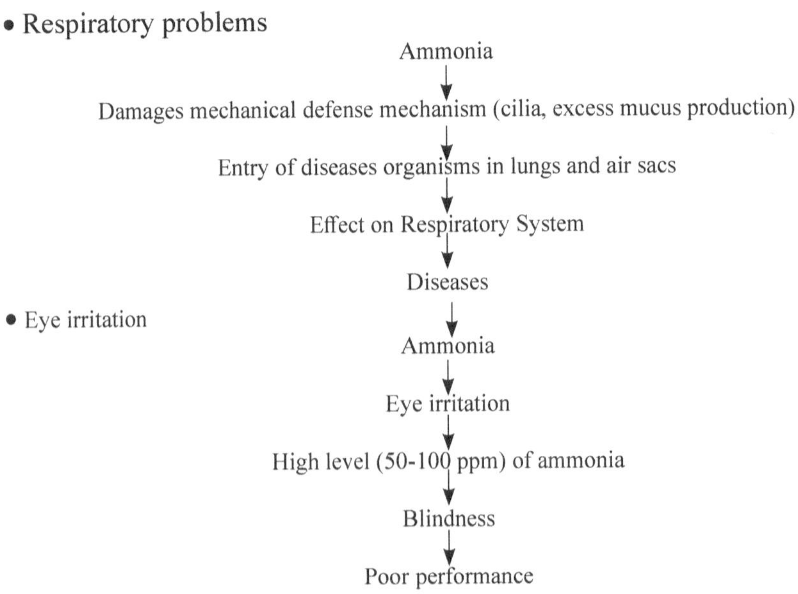

Other Potential Hazards

- Burnt foot pads and skin and leg problems.
- Breast blisters, breast buttons and scabby areas.
- Bruising, condemnations and downgrading of carcass
- Coccidia sporulation – younger birds
- *E. coli*, CRD, Brooder pneumonia.
- Increased Fly population.

Prevention or Control

- Use fresh and good quality litter material
- To ensure proper drying, please make sure to rake the litter at least twice a day.
- Please rake the area using a scoop to break up any clumps thoroughly.
- Attention all poultry farmers! For optimal hygiene, we recommend that you always rake the litter in layers after egg collection. This simple step will help ensure the health of your flock and the quality of your eggs. Don't let dirty litter compromise your operation - make sure to prioritize cleanliness today!
- Proper ventilation to remove excess moisture.
- Change the location of waterer frequently.
- Proper medication to prevent diarrhea (for any reason).
- Frequently remove wet/caked litter especially around waterers and feeders.
- Change wet litter with fresh dried ones.
- Addition of hydrated lime powder @ 1 kg or super phosphate of lime @ 0.75 kg per sq. m can be used which act as water absorbent.
- A mixture of wood ash and superphosphate in a ratio of 4:1 can also be used.
- Higher temperature and overcrowding also can predispose to wet-litter.
- By raising the floor 0.3 to 0.5 meters above ground level, we have taken proactive measures to prevent any water seepage. This ensures that you can rest easy knowing that your space is protected from any potential water damage.
- Overhangs to the roof must be adequate to protect interior of the house from rain water.

Conclusion

Maintaining appropriate moisture levels in poultry house litter is crucial for optimal flock production. Provide good feed, prevent disease, ensure ventilation, and use quality bedding.

16

Quality Control for Poultry and Livestock Feed

Om Prakash Dinani

Poultry Science Department
College of Veterinary Science & A.H. Anjora, Durg
Dau Shri Vasudev Chandrakar Kamdhenu Vishwavidyalaya
Durg, Chhattisgarh

Most raw feed ingredients used as an energy and/or a protein source in poultry feed are grown, harvested, processed, and transported from outside of the poultry industry. Poultry feed are routinely subjected to contamination from diverse sources which may have a serious consequences on the safety of poultry products. Public concerns over food safety from the food of animal origin is a cause of global concern in the recent years due to problems such as bovine spongiform encephalopathy (BSE), dioxin and melamine contaminations, microbial resistance to antibiotics and outbreak of food borne bacterial infections (food poisoning) (Panda, 2013). The contaminants enter into the body system by consumption of contaminated poultry products and thereby producing adverse effect on human health. Some of the potential feed contamination sources in poultry feed in all most all production systems are microbial agents, chemical contaminations and mycotoxins (fungal toxins). These agents may contaminate the poultry feed at any stage of production till up-to the point of feeding and may have adverse effect on poultry and affects human health upon consumption of such contaminated food of poultry origin (egg or meat).

World food and feed demands are increasing due to increase in human, livestock and poultry population along with increase demand of biofuel. Poverty, food and nutrition insecurity are intrinsically linked. About 70% global compounded feed went to monogastric animals (Steinfeld *et al.*,2010). Poultry & Livestock supply 16% of the energy and 28-35% protein consumed globally. Food and feed quality are important due to harmful residual effect of chemicals connected by food chain. (FAO, 2009; IAASTD, 2009 and Steinfeld *et.al*, 2010). A billion extra tonnes of grain needed to satisfy future food, feed, and fuel demands (IAASTD, 2009).Poultry/Animals convert low-biological-value protein foods that are less palatable and less nutrient dense to high-biological-value foods that are highly palatable and nutrient dense.

Mycotoxins Contamination of Feed

Mycotoxin in feed are considered to be the second most serious issues in poultry industry following increased feed price. Mycotoxins are the toxins produced by different fungus on agricultural products during harvest, transportation or storage. Mycotoxins are produced readily in groundnuts, corn, cottonseed, feedstuffs derived from these commodities, and a variety of other cereal grains and oilseeds (Dhavan and Choudary, 1995). When feed contaminated with mycotoxins are consumed by the bird, mycotoxicosis occurs. Mycotoxicosis is the most devastating and wide spread non infectious disease affecting all species of livestock and poultry (all breeds and all age group of poultry). It is more common in tropical countries like India, especially in areas of hot and humid climatic conditions, leading to great economic loss. Among the poultry species ducklings are more susceptible followed by turkey, poults, pheasants, chicks, mature chicken and quail in that order.

If not stored properly, poultry feed ingredients as well as mixed feed get infected by bacteria and fungi. Among these, fungal infestation with *Aspergillus, Penicillium* and *Fusarium* which liberates highly toxic mycotoxins as secondary metabolites is a common experience in the field. In the course of their development, fungi also utilize the feed nutrients, contributing to a reduction in their content and also reduce the organoleptic quality of the feed. The environment plays an important role in fungal infestation. Conditions like high humidity, moderate to high temperature, higher grain moisture content, improper harvest and storage favours the development of these fungi of the host substrate are major determining environmental factors in fungal infestation. Fungi can infect the feed ingredients either in the field itself or any stage between the harvest and ingestion by the bird.

Favourable condition for growth of fungi

Environmental conditions	Levels
Moisture	12-14% or higher
Relative humidity in the go-down	Above 70-75%
Physical condition of the grain	Damaged seed coat due to insects and improper harvesting
Ambient temperature	Moderate to high (25-30°C) for *Aspergillus*
	Low (15-20°C) for *Fusarium*
Storage	Leaky roof in the go-down and moist floor
	Improper stacking of bags and poor ventilation

When grown on the feed, the fungi produce secondary toxic metabolites called mycotoxins. Fungi that produce mycotoxins of major significance in the poultry are *Apergillus*, *Fusarium* and *Penicillium*. *Aspergillus* and *Penicillum* are a common problem in the stored feed ingredients whereas *Fusarium* is basically a field fungus and affects the grain before being harvested (Williams *et al.*, 2004). Though hundreds of mycotoxins have been identified in feedstuffs, the mycotoxins of practical importance to poultry include aflatoxin, ochratoxin, T-2toxin, citrinin, deoxynivalenol, fumonisins and zearalenone.

Major Fungi genera with associated mycotoxins

Fungi genera	**Associated Mycotoxins**
Aspergillus	Aflatoxin, Ochratoxin, Cyclopiazonic acid, Citrinin
Penicillum	Ochratoxin, Citrinin, Cyclopiazonic acid, Penicillic acid
Fusarium	Fumonisins, Moniliformin, Zearalenone, Deoxynivalenol, Nivalenol, T-2Toxin, Fusaric acid
Claviceps	Ergot alkaloids

Aflatoxin is the most commonly occurring mycotoxins in India and is produced by the fungi *Aspergillus flavus* and *Aspergillus parasiticus (*Dutta and Das, 2001*)*. It is commonly seen in maize, jowar, groundnut cake, coconut cake, cottonseed cake/meal and mixed feed (Dhavan and Choudary, 1995). There are a number of distinct but structurally related aflatoxin compounds but the four most commonly noticed are B1, B2, G1 and G2. Amongst these, aflatoxin B1 is the most common and most toxic compounds present in the contaminated feed samples. Aflatoxin produces adverse effect in poultry resulting in decreased immunity even leading to death (Sravanan *et al.*, 2006). After being exposed to aflatoxin contaminated feed birds develop anorexia, listlessness, poor FCR, decreased body weight, immunosuppression and susceptibility to stress (Leeson *et al.*, 1995). Aflatoxin is a hepato toxin causing liver hypertrophy, paleness and fatty degeneration of liver (Ledous *et al.*, 1999).

Ochratoxin is the second major mycotoxins prevalent in poultry feed after aflatoxin in India. It is produced by the fungi *Aspergillus ochraceus* and *Penicillium viridicatum* at a wide range of environmental conditions (temperature, 4-37°C and moisture content, 18-40%) (Hessltine *et al.*, 1972). It is commonly found in barley, maize, wheat, jowar, bajra, groundnuts and sunflower extractions and mixed feed (Chandrasekaran, 1996). There are mainly two types of ochratoxin (A and B) and ochratoxin A is more ubiquitous than ochratoxin B. Ochratoxin has teratogenic, mutagenic and immune-toxic effects (Huff *et al.*, 1974) in livestock and poultry.

Depending on the degree of contamination, mycotoxins or their metabolites, may be deposited in the poultry products like egg and meat. Though, the concentrations in poultry products are considerably lower than the levels present in the feed and may not cause acute toxicity in human, but residues of carcinogenic mycotoxins such as aflatoxins and ochratoxin A can affect human health. A frequently asked question is what is the safe levels of different mycotoxins in poultry feed? As described earlier dietary mycotoxins depend on a number of factors for producing its toxicity, it is difficult to spell out correctly the safe levels. However, under optimal managemental conditions levels of 20-30 ppb aflatoxin, 50-70 ppb ochratoxin and 100 ppb T-2 toxin may be considered safe for poultry on short term feeding. Prevention and control of mycotoxin contamination

In general, mycotoxins are relatively stable compounds that are not destroyed by processing of feed and may even be concentrated by screening. Poultry feed, if excessively contaminated with mycotoxins (beyond the permissible levels), it should not be fed to the birds producing eggs or meat for human consumption.

Prevention

Mycotoxins are, in general, very stable compounds remaining intact in stored grains for long periods. The best approach to control mycotoxin production in feedstuff is to prevent fungi growth. Mycotoxins contamination can be prevented by following strict measures like

- Proper storage of raw materials and mixed feeds
- Moisture levels should be below the minimum threshold levels (<12%)
- Maintaining proper relative humidity in the go-down (<60%)
- Ideal temperature during storage in the go-down (<15°C)
- Proper ventilation in the go-down
- Protecting against insects and rodents during storage
- Proper processing
- Addition of antifungal compounds during storage

Control

Many strategies have been attempted in the past to counteract the adverse effect of mycotoxins on poultry health and production. Some of the mycotoxin binders (adsorbents) extensively studied in poultry is activated charcoal, hydroxyl sodium calcium aluminosilicate (HSCAC), bentonites, zeolites etc (Dalvi and Mcgowan, 1984; Ramakrishna *et al.*, 1992; Scheideler *et al.*, 1993). It has been reported that HSCAC and Na-bentonite can adsorb and retain upto

95% aflatoxin. Mannanoligosaccharide (MOS) is derived from the cell wall of yeast *Saccharomyces cerevisiae*, has the ability to bind several pathogens in the gastrointestinal tract and thereby prevent their colonization (Mahesh and Devegowda, 1996, Raju and Devegowda, 2000). It has been reported that MOS can binds with AFB1 and zearalenone and AFB1. It has also been suggested that addition of dietary esterified glucomannan is effective in broilers to counteract *in vivo* toxic effects of feed naturally contaminated with AF, ochratoxin, zearalenone, and T-2 toxin (Aravind *et al.*, 2003). Organic acids have long been used to inhibit mould growth and mycotoxin development in stored in raw materials and methods. Organic acids such as propionic acid and formic acid are effective inhibitors (Martin *et al.*, 2000). It has been reported that supplementation of vitamin C, E and Se reduces the damage caused by mycotoxins such as DON and T-2toxin to liver.

Chemical Contamination of Feed

Various chemicals such as veterinary drugs (antibiotics/coccidiostats), agricultural (pesticides/ fungicides), industrial (dioxin), heavy metals (lead/ mercury/cadmium) and adulterants (melamine) may enter into the poultry feed. When such contaminated feed is fed to the bird, the chemicals can accumulate in tissues or incorporated into the eggs and cause health problems in humans.

Antibiotics are routinely used as feed additives by the poultry industry and poultry veterinarians to enhance growth and feed efficiency and reduce the incidence of disease. No doubt, antibiotic usage has facilitated the efficient production of poultry, allowing the consumer to purchase egg and meat at a reasonable cost. Antibiotic usage has also enhanced the health and well-being of poultry by reducing the incidence of disease (Jones and Ricke, 2003). However, the possible development of microbial resistance to the use of antimicrobial in poultry feed has become a major public concern in recent years (Panda *et al.*, 2009). As a result the routine use of antibiotics as feed additives is either banned or restricted in the poultry industries in many developed countries.

Although some antibiotics are approved for use in poultry, there is extensive regulatory oversight to ensure the safety of foods from poultry origin. However, in the developing countries like India, still the poultry industry is relying heavily on antibiotics. This could be due to lack of proper bio-security measures in the production system followed. Some of the antimicrobial compounds approved for use in broiler feeds without a veterinary prescription (Miller, 2001) have given in the Table below. If antibiotics are used in broiler feed, it is always recommend providing a withdrawal period (7-10 days) prior to slaughter to overcome problem of drug residues in meat and should be used judiciously. In a consumer survey, it was reported that 77% of consumers responding considered animal drug residues in meats be an extreme health concern (Donoghue, 2003). Today, in USA, the Food and Drug Administration strictly regulate the use of anti-microbial and the USDA to warrant their safety and efficacy.

A variety of chemicals (weedicides, insecticides, fungicides and rodenticides) have been used in modern agriculture and animal husbandry practices and residues of these chemicals or their metabolites may remain in the plant crops or animal foods at concentrations that may be hazardous to the consumers. Again, during the journey from the production site to the consumer place, food commodities are exposed to multitude hazards that may lead to contamination by dust, weeds, mechanical injury, physical changes accelerated by heat, light, contamination or spoilage due to microorganisms, insects and rodents or biochemical changes brought about by enzymes that may be endogenous or contributed by the invading biological agents. Thus food commodities are likely to undergo significant alterations. To prevent such alterations again the food commodities are treated with chemicals (insecticides and pesticides).

Antimicrobial compounds approved for use in broiler feeds without a veterinary prescription (Miller, 2001)

Drug name	**Indications for use**	**Human use**
Amprolium	Coccidiosis	None
Arsanilic acid	Growth promotion, feed efficiency	None
Bacitracin methylene disalicylate	Rate of weight gain, feed efficiency	None
Bacitracin zinc	Rate of weight gain, feed efficiency	Yes
Bambermycins	Rate of weight gain, feed efficiency	None
Decoquinate	Coccidiosis	None
Diclazuril	Coccidiosis	None
Erythromycin	Prevention of infectious coryza	Yes
Halofuginone hydrobromide	Coccidiosis	None
Hygromycin B	Worms	None
Lasalocid	Coccidiosis	None
Linomycin	Rate of weight gain, feed efficiency	Yes
Maduramicin ammonium	Coccidiosis	None
Monensin	Coccidiosis	None
Narasin	Coccidiosis	None
Narasin/ nicarbazin	Coccidiosis	None
Nicarbazin	Coccidiosis	None
Nitarsone	Blackhead	None
Novobiocin	Stapylococcus infections	Yes
Salinomycin	Coccidiosis	None

Drug name	Indications for use	Human use
Semduramicin	Coccidiosis	None
Sulfadimethoxine and ormetroprim 5:3	Coccidiosis	None
Tylosin	Rate of weight gain, feed efficiency	None
Virginiamycin	Rate of weight gain, feed efficiency	None

Insecticides and Pesticides

India is one of the largest producers and consumers of insecticides and pesticides in South Asia and use of pesticides have been on the rise in the last three decades (Venkatraman, 1992). In our country insecticides and pesticides have become an important tool for boosting production and proper storage of feed ingredients. During the first four decades of the 20th century (1900-1940), use of insecticides and pesticides was limited to few simple compounds (Bordeaur-fungicide, dintro-orthocresol-herbicide & insecticides and sodium chlorate-herbicide). However, after the second world war, research in pesticide chemistry increased rapidly and organochloro and organophosphorus insecticides were discovered. During the last three decades a wide range of more complex chemicals have been developed and also the consumption pattern has changed. Prevention and control of contaminants and pesticides in the poultry production requires knowledge of the sources of contamination and their consequences and also the knowledge of possibilities to exclude these sources from the system or to reduce the effect.

The presence of insecticides and pesticide, and contaminants in the feed of poultry not only depressed their productive performance but also lead to accumulation of their residues in the different organs is a major public health concern from consumer points of view. Therefore a holistic approach is needed for judicious and careful use of insecticides and pesticide in the plant right from the production sites till it reaches the animal or bird not only from the bird's health arena but also the consumers concern.

Dioxins

Dioxins are group polychlorinated aromatic compounds (organic compound) which are colourless, odourless containing carbon, hydrogen, oxygen and chlorine. The term dioxin refers to a broad family of chemicals. Of the 210 different dioxin compounds, only 17 are of toxicological concern. The most widely studied and most toxic form of dioxin is 2,3,7,8-tetrachlorodibenzo-p-dioxin, abbreviated as 2,3,7,8-TCDD. They are not produced intentionally or deliberately, but are formed as a by-product of chemical processes. These range from natural events such as volcano eruptions and forest fires to man- made processes such as manufacturing of chemicals, pesticides, steel and paints, pulp and paper bleaching, exhaust emissions and incineration (Kan, 2002). For example, when chlorinated waste is burned in an uncontrolled way in an incinerator, the emissions to the air contain dioxins. Dioxins are not soluble in water and are highly soluble in fat. They bind to sediment and organic matter in the environment and are absorbed in animal and human fatty tissue. In addition they are not biodegradable so they are persistent and bio-accumulate in the food chain (Kan, 2002). This means that once released into the environment, via air or via water, they pile up in the fat tissue of animals and humans. Soil is a natural sink for dioxins. Apart from atmospheric deposition, soil may be polluted by sewage sludge or composts, pills and erosion from nearby contaminated areas. Soil is absorbed, directly or indirectly via dust deposits on vegetables, by free-range grazing cattle, goats, sheep and chicken. Pirard and de Pauw (2006; 2007) have reported carry-over of chlorinated dioxins and furans as well as brominated diphenyl ethers in laying hens from feed to egg.

Melamine

Melamine is a by-product of the coal industry. Melamine is a synthetically produced chemical used for a wide variety of applications, including plastics, adhesives, laminates, paints, permanent- press fabrics, flame retardants, textile finishes, tarnish inhibitors, paper coatings and fertilizer mixtures. Melamine (1,3,5-triazine-2,4,6-triamine) is high in nitrogen (C3N6H6). Melamine is added to protein supplements used in feeds such as wheat gluten, maize gluten and rice gluten to artificially inflate protein levels. Melamine may also enter the food-chain indirectly through animal feeds that have been treated with products containing melamine, such as fertilizers or pesticides/herbicides. In 2007, the adulteration of pet-food with melamine leads to the death of hundreds of cats and dogs in the USA (Science Daily, 2007). This also triggered the testing of other animal feed for melamine and low levels of melamine were found in feed for fish, poultry and pigs. Regulation regarding its use in animal feed do not always exists as it is only recent events which indicated the need to regulate for this substance. However, some countries have established regulations and do not permit the use of melamine in animal feed.

Heavy Metals

One of the important features of heavy metals is that the chemical form in which they are present may change during passage through the intestine or storage in animal tissue, but they are not metabolized. Beihl and Buck (1987) reported that excessive amounts of metals in animal feed and feedstuffs are often due to human actions. Some important contaminants are cadmium, lead and mercury as well as arsenic, although the latter is by definition not a heavy metal. The contamination of heavy metals in poultry feed can be avoided by not including the contaminated feedstuffs. However, environmental and incidental exposure is hard to control. The checks on levels of heavy metals in animal products are generally conducted on a survey basis and prevention of occurrence of products with volatile levels of heavy metals seldom or never occurs (Kan, 2002).

Microbial Contamination of Feed

The major cause of concern in poultry feed is *Salmonella* which is associated with food poisoning in humans (Cliver and Rieman, 2002). Salmonella is widely distributed in nature and poultry feed may be a source of *Salmonella* contamination. One potential source of *Salmonella* contamination of poultry feed is fish meal. The use of fish meal has been restricted in many countries because of possible contamination with microbes such as *Salmonella and Escherichia.* The contamination of poultry feed by *Salmonella* can be avoided by using feedstuffs free of *Salmonella* while diet formulation.

Most raw feed ingredients used as an energy and/or a protein source in poultry feed are grown, harvested, processed, and transported from outside of the poultry industry. Therefore, the ingredient quality control is an important first step in preventing the contamination of birds on the farm. Serotyping becomes very important when tracing the origin of a *Salmonella* infection in animals, especially humans. For example, it is well known that *Salmonella* can be transmitted from feed ingredients to the completed mixed feed and on to live poultry. This transmission sometimes results in the production of *Salmonella*-positive products (i.e., meat and eggs). Many times the *Salmonella* serotypes found in feed ingredients are not the same as those commonly found in processed poultry. An integrated Hazard Analysis and Critical Control Point (HACCP) program is essential to eliminate *Salmonella* from poultry industry.

Transgenic Feed for Poultry

Biotech/ transgenic crops are similar to their traditional counterparts, but they have been engineered to possess special characteristics that make them better. These crops are for the benefit of both farmers and consumers with higher crop yields and with the use of less chemical inputs. The introduction of genetically modified crops in 1996 for herbicide tolerance has consistently been the dominant trait followed by insect resistance. Foreign genes were successfully introduced into plants for the first time 30 years ago. Genetically modified (GM) crops came up with a promise of a second green revolution, deliver profits to farmers and promote a greener environment. Crops engineered to carry useful traits now grow on 170 million hectares in at least 28 countries. The market is mainly dominated by a few insect-resistant and herbicide-tolerant crops. The environmental benefits have been a dispute, and activists question the safety of GM foods. The number of countries growing biotech crops has increased from 6 in 1996, the first year of commercialization, to 18 in 2003 and 25 in 2008. The top eight countries growing more than one million hectares of biotech crops are; USA (62.5 million hectares), Argentina (21.0), Brazil (15.8), India (7.6), Canada (7.6), China (3.8), Paraguay (2.7), and South Africa (1.8 million hectares). In 2008, 5 million small farmers planted 7.6 million hectares of Bt cotton as cotton being the major biotech crop in India (www.isaaa.org). The major importance of GM crops is their capability to contribute to: 1) Increasing crop productivity; 2) Land-saving technology capable; 3) More efficient use of external inputs: 4) Increasing stability of production and 5) to improve the economic and social benefits.

The GM crops are used directly as animal feed such as maize, rice, sorghum etc. or as their byproducts from the processing industries such as meals, bran, cakes, distiller grain, etc. Thus there is need for nutritional and safety assessment of feeds from GMO in origin. The safety and nutritional studies with feeds from GM crops in origin have been reviewed (Aumaitre *et al.*, 2002; Chesson and Flachowsky, 2003; Clark and Ipharraguerre, 2001).

Comparison of transgenic and isogenic feed ingredients in chicken

Transgenic Feed Ingredient	**Chemical composition**	**Performance of broiler/ layer**	**Source**
Bt Maize	Similar	Higher gain in BT group	Piva *et al.*, 2001
Herbicide tolerant	Similar	Similar	Sidhu *et al.*, 2000
Maize			
Herbicide tolerant soybean meal	Similar	Similar	Hammond *et al.*, 1996
Bt Cotton	Similar	Similar	Elangovan *et al.*, 2002; Mandal *et al.*, 2004; Elangovan *et al.*, 2006
Bt Potato	Similar	Similar	Halle *et al.*, 2005
Bt Brinjal	Similar	Similar	Shrivastava *et al.*, 2006
Bt Rice	Similar	Similar	Tyagi *et al.*, 2011
Bt Corn	Similar	Similar	Tyagi *et al.*, 2011

Feed Safety Guidelines

National Organizations

a. **AGMARK (1973)-**Quality certification mark. Voluntary regulation

b. **PFA act (1954)**-Now FSSAI (2006)-Mandatory regulation.

c. **BIS act** (1986)-Voluntary regulation
   - H.Q.-New Delhi
   - Ministry of consumer affairs, Food & Public distribution
   - also works as WTO-TBT enquiry point for India
   - Published more than 19000 std.
   - also undertaking HACCP certification.

d. **HACCP certification-** Voluntary regulation
   - It is a food safety system.
   - It is minimum std. for trade.
   - It focuses on physical, chemical and microbiological hazards.
   - It is modern concept of quality management for food items

e. **Other food safety management system-**

f. **GHP/GMP** (Health/manufacturing)

g. **CLFMA-** Voluntary guideline to follow feed safety.

h. **APEDA-** All EOU mandatory have HACCP and ISO std. as per APEDA

International Organizations

a. ISO,1947- 89 countries are members

b. ISO 9000 series applicable for both manufacturing and service industry

c. CAC,1963 by FAO & WHO-for uniform std.

d. **USA-** FDA, AAFCO (Association of American feed control officials)
   - Voluntary membership
   - Surveillance system for animal feed for microbial contamination
   - HACCP Programme-7 principles
   - Salmonella negative std. for animal feed

e. **EU-** European feed safety authority
   - Risk management for animal feed
   - Strong enforcement

f. **USA- FDA, AAFCO** (Association of American feed control officials)
   - Voluntary membership
   - Surveillance system for animal feed for microbial contamination
   - HACCP Programme-7 principles
   - Salmonella negative std. for animal feed

g. **EU**- European feed safety authority
   - Risk management for animal feed
   - Strong enforcement

Quality Control of Feed Ingredients

Qualitative test-Physical analysis/Analyst's skill. Colour/odour/texture/ particle size/shape/wetting/adulterations-Husk/sand/limestone Physical changes-colour/odour/mold growth

Methods-

a. Winnowing/Air blowing-To detect husk
b. Soaking- To detect sand
c. Sieving-particle size

Quantities test-Chemical analysis

Proximate principles, NIRS, AOAC methods, TLC, HPLC, AAS

Chemical changes-gelatinization, Maillard reaction, rancidity

ANF

a. Extrinsic-weeds/insecticides
b. Intrinsic-SBM-trypsin inhibitors/urease

Protein quality-Protein/nitrogen solubility, FDNB, Pepsin / AA digestibility

Microscopic evaluation

- Used for identifying & confirming adulterants/feed ingredients (AOAC,1970)
- Adulterants/feed ingredients studied under low/high magnification
- Low (8X-50X)-Physical analysis
- High (100X-500X)-Plant cell & structural features, grinded feed

Table 1: Scale of Sample (BIS)

Lot Size	No. of bags to b e selected
Up to 50	5
51-100	8
101-300	13
301-500	22
501 and above	32

Table 2: Common Adulterants

S. No.	Feed Ingredients	Adulterants
1.	GNC	GNC husk, urea, non-edible oil cake
2.	SBM	Urea, raw soybean
3.	Mustard cake	*Argimona maxicina* seeds, fibrous feed ingredients, urea
4.	DORB	Rice huk, saw dust
5.	Fish meal (*Salmonella* and *Escherichia*) source	Salt, urea, sand
6.	Mineral Mixture	Salt, sand, limestone, marble powder
7.	Mollasses	Water
8.	Maize	Cobs
9.	Rice kanki	Stone particles, marble, lime stone

Table 3: Use of Damaged Food Grains: As Per Quality Control Manual of FCI (5 categories)

Class	Sound/slightly damage/touched & broken grain %	Category for which declared fit
Feed 1	70-85	Poultry/pig
Feed 2	55-70	Ruminants
Feed 3	30-55	Industrial
Mature	10-30	Manure
Dumping	4-10	Dumping

Table 4: BIS specification for only chicken feed & M.M. are available, But Not For Other Poultry Sp.; However ICAR- CARI Has Given Many Such Specification of Different Poultry Sp. Along With Specification For Many Feed Ingredients

Quality Parameter of chicken feed (BIS)	Max.%
1.Moisture	11
2.AIA	4.5
3.CF	10
4.Salt	0.5
5.Aflatoxin	20 ppb

Conclusions

The genetic manipulation has produced a number of new transgenic varieties of commodity crops with desirable features, such as protection against common pests, tolerance to herbicides, and improved nutritional quality characteristics. Trials with poultry, catfish, swine, cattle and sheep have demonstrated that feeds derived from transgenic crop plants are equivalent to conventional crops in safety and feed value. Commercial formulations of such Bt-based products have been registered for use on food crops in the US since 1961. However, questions regarding the digestive fate of DNA and protein from transgenic plants have been raised in regard to human consumption and trade of animal products e.g., meat, milk, and eggs from animals fed transgenic crops. In addition to feed safety assessment, including safety for consumers, animals and environment, nutritional assessment of feeds produced using recombinant DNA techniques is necessary and should be considered as an essential part of safety assessment.

Some of the possible approaches (Panda, 2004) in on the use of insecticides and pesticides is as follows:

- Strict legislation on the use of insecticides and pesticides during either production or storage of feed ingredients
- Judicious use of less persistent and biodegradable synthetic pesticides
- Use of bio-pesticides as it is safer to Humans and do not leave any toxic residues in the crops as well as environment
- Integrated pest management and integrated nutrient management technique
- Organic farming– It is gaining popularity now a days as it produce environment healthy safe food. It also maintains soil fertility and control of pest and diseases are achieved through enhancement of biological and ecological interactions.

The quality of ingredients used for making poultry feed is important because what birds eat can affect flock quality and the wholesomeness of poultry products such as meat and egg. Feed safety and its regulations are thus of major international concern in poultry production. Most raw feed ingredients used in poultry feed are grown, harvested, processed, and transported from outside of the poultry industry. Carryover of toxic substances from feed to food is influenced by absorption, metabolism and excretion of the compounds. The ingredient quality control is an important first step in preventing the contamination of birds on the farm. The direct links between feed safety and the safety of foods of poultry origin is well established. Therefore, it is essential that the feed production and manufacture procedures need to meet the stringent safety requirements. In spite of large numbers of published information on residues in products of animal origin and carry-over of toxic substances, specific knowledge on the dynamics of turnover in bird is scarce. Information on possible intervention strategies as a risk management tool to be used in a HACCP approach is often lacking. Development of quality systems in existing circumstances requires this knowledge and warrants further research.

- Mandatory regulations are needed, not voluntary for feed safety
- Establishment of strong regulatory body for enforcement of regulations (Like FSSAI)
- Establishment of reference & central laboratory for animal/poultry feed analysis and quantifying the harmful chemical residues
- Packaged livestock feed should be certified for quality assurance, should mention the nutrient composition, packaging date and best before date.
- Sun-drying and processing of feed is effective way to minimize microbiological hazard.
- Reuse of gunny bags should be avoided.
- FCI-C Processing of food/feed should be encouraged to increase keeping quality.
- Effective rodent control programme and IPM.
- On spot test needed to be developed to identify hazards.
- Use of bio-pesticide & bio-fertilizers to minimize chemical residues.
- Encourage Organic farming.
- Revision of regulation for GM/Transgenic crops.
- WC and SWC should be as per requirement & upgraded.
- Food processing and preservation techniques for food security and increased nutrient availability at the household level.
- Uniting food, health and nutrition in Agricultural Research. (One Health concept)
- Advocacy for Agricultural policies to incorporate nutritional objectives.
- Advocacy for Health policies with agricultural and nutrition considerations.
- The key message is action to implement and scale up known solutions.

17

Rare Earth Elements in Poultry Nutrition

Bhaisare D.B.[1], Kadam, M.M.[1], Pawar, O.K.[1], Aswathi, P.B.[2] and Bokade, H.S.[1]

[1]*Department of Poultry Science, Nagpur Veterinary College, Nagpur Maharashtra*
[2]*Department of Poultry Science, College of Veterinary and Animal Sciences Pookode, Wayanad, Kerala*

Introduction

The rare-earth elements (REEs) consist of a group of 17 elements that have atomic numbers between 57 (lanthanum) and 71 (lutetium). They are also known as lanthanides. The European Union banned all in-feed growth-promoting antibiotics in 2006 because of public fears about the transmission and development of multi-resistant bacteria, which pose a threat to human health. Such restrictions have prompted the need to explore new safe, efficient, and inexpensive feed additives as alternative sources of growth promoters. Rare earth elements (REEs) have been used as feed additives for the last few decades due to their effectiveness in improving the body weight, feed conversion rate (FCR), and milk and egg production in various farm animals, including cattle, poultry, and swine. He *et al.* (2010) noted that REEs have the potential to become new natural feed additives that can enhance animal performance. Rare earth elements are grouped together with metallic elements that share similar properties. Scandium, yttrium, lanthanum, cerium, praseodymium, neodymium, promethium, samarium, europium, gadolinium, terbium, dysprosium, holmium, erbium, thulium, ytterbium, and lutetium are rare earth elements called lanthanides (Richter *et al.*, 2006).

History

An unusual black rock was discovered by a miner in Ytterby, Sweden in 1788. In 1794, it was discovered as a new kind of 'earth', which is a reference to acid-soluble elements from ancient times (Rowlatt, 2014). Later, it was discovered to be a mineral that consists of cerium, lanthanum, and yttrium in iron ore. It was later found to be a mineral consisting of cerium, lanthanum and yttrium in iron ore. Because these elements were not found elsewhere, they were assumed to be scarce. Hence the name, rare T earths. In 1803, Cerium was isolated first, while Lutetium was last isolated in 1907. The term rare earth elements consists of scandium (21), yttrium (39), lanthanum (57), and the 14 chemical elements that follow lanthanum (58 -71) called lanthanoids. Due to their chemical and physical similarities with the lanthanides, Scandium (atomic number 21) and Yttrium (atomic number 39) are also classified as rare-earth elements. The majority of them are found in the Earth's crust (Redling, 2006) and contain group III elements from the periodic table, including cerium (Ce), lanthanum (La), scandium (Sc), yttrium (Y), and 14 La-like elements called lanthanoids (IUPAC, 2005). Despite being found in nature, rare-earth elements cannot be found in pure metal form and the rarest, due to the absence of long-lived or stable isotopes, promethium is only found in trace amounts in natural materials (Castor and Hendrik, 2006). The average concentration of rare earth elements in the Earth's crust is estimated to be between 130 and 240 mg/g, which is significantly higher than other metals.

Mechanisms of Action

Ou *et al.* (2000) proposed four potential mechanisms for REE, which included increased enzyme activity, enhanced protein metabolism, suppression of bacterial growth, and promotion of digestive fluid secretion in the stomach. Flachowski (2003) proposes that REEs can promote growth in animals through their anti-inflammatory and immunostimulant effects. Additionally, REEs may have effects on hormone activity and cell proliferation that could enhance their effects (He *et al.*, 2010). Despite numerous studies examining the mechanisms behind REE-enhanced ruminal degradability of feeds, they remain unclear. Monogastric animals have been extensively studied to investigate the possible mechanisms of action of REEs in the digestive tract. Ou *et al.* (2000) concluded by inducing digestive enzymes in the intestine and destroying infectious bacteria, REE supplementation can enhance nutrient digestion and absorption. REEs have recently been reported to have antibacterial properties by selectively inhibiting the growth of specific bacteria species in the digestive system. *Zhang et al.* (2000) and Peng *et al.* (2004) observed that REEs had a dose-dependent effect on suppressing the growth of certain bacteria. Similarly, REEs can modulate digestive microorganisms and enzymes (Xun *et al.*, 2014). The mechanistic actions of REEs were profound about high nutrient absorption and enhanced digestive enzyme secretions, hence enhancing growth performance and the process of digestion (Azer, 2003).

Biological Applications

They exhibit antibacterial, anticoagulant, cytotoxic, and phosphate-binding properties. However, most of their actions are attributed to their impact on Ca2+dependent pathways, which may also play a role in specific medical conditions. Since they supply different radioisotopes that radiate in the α, β, or γ-range. A few of them even have paramagnetic characteristics. They are now helpful for luminous biomarker and anticancer diagnosis and treatment (Townley, 2013). Rare earths are added to animal feed in addition to being utilized as fertilizers for plants in agriculture. Due to their strong attraction for ionic bonding and preference for the tripositive oxidation state, rare earths can produce a wide variety of rare earth salts, both organic and inorganic. However, rare earths can also combine to create complexes, particularly when chelating oxygen ligands are included. Rare earth elements can be found in several minerals found in nature, including monazite and bastnaesite, which are primarily utilized in industrial processes. Rare earth elements are now found in many commonly used electronics, including computers, televisions, and lighters. They can also be found in aerospace, nuclear engineering, medical technology, the automotive sector, and military equipment. Additionally, medications containing rare earth elements are used to treat burns and hyperphosphatemia in individuals with chronic renal failure. Rare earths may be used in organ transplantation, osteoporosis and atherosclerosis treatment and prevention, and cancer treatments in the future, among other applications. For many years, China has effectively utilized rare earth elements as fertilizers and feed additives at low percentages. attained in a variety of plant species, including fruits, vegetables, and cereals, following the application of rare earth.

Use as Feed Additives in Animals

Rare earths have been demonstrated to increase feed conversion and body weight gain in almost all types of farming animals when added to feed (chickens, pigs, ducks, cattle). Improvements were also observed in the amount of milk produced by dairy cows, the number of eggs laid by laying hens, the output and survival rate of fish, and the pace at which shrimp eggs hatch. As a result, feed additives containing light rare earths (La, Ce, Pr, Nd) are typically employed. Although commercially available rare earth feed additives can be found in both organic and inorganic forms (nitrates, chlorides, etc.), organic forms are said to yield superior results. Results from investigations on the impact of rare earths on plant growth have been contentious, however some animal feeding trials in the West have shown that dietary rare earth application significantly enhances performance. Pigs fed diets supplemented with low-dose rare earth chlorides showed improvements in feed conversion rate of 10% and body weight growth of up to 19%. However, after rare earth citrates were added to the pigs' diet, even better results were observed. Results from investigations on the impact of rare earths on plant growth have been contentious, however some animal feeding trials in the West have shown that dietary rare earth application significantly enhances performance. Pigs fed diets supplemented with low-dose rare earth chlorides showed improvements in feed conversion rate of 10% and body weight growth of up to 19%. However, after rare earth citrates were added to the pigs' diet, even better results were observed (Evans, 1990; Xie and Wang,1998; He *et al.*,1999).

Use as Feed Additives in Aoultry

There have reportedly been several findings on the growth-promoting impact of REE in poultry published in the literature, particularly in Chinese literature (Igbasan*et al.*, 2012). It was discovered that adding 200, 400, 600, and 800 mg/kg REE to the food considerably enhanced the number of eggs produced and their weight in laying hens (Wu *et al.*, 1994). The impact of feeding 53-week-old laying hens diets supplemented with 300, 400, and 500 mg/kg of REE-nitrate was investigated by Zhang *et al* (1996). The outcome demonstrated a substantial ($P < 0.05$) improvement in laying rate with diets containing 300 and 400 mg/kg of REE.Ca2+ is essential for many different physiological and metabolic functions in both human and animal systems. Rare earth elements are especially used to substitute Ca2+ in a variety of biological processes since they are similar to calcium in terms of size, bonding, coordination geometry, and donor atom preference. Because it is necessary for the creation of the egg and a member of the signaling system that influences oviduct, gastrointestinal, and nervous system motility, calcium is significant in egg production. 400 mg/kg of dietary lanthanum oxide supplementation dramatically ($P<0.05$) increased body mass (Durmus *et al.*, 2015).

Rare earths have also been demonstrated to improve feed conversion by up to 3% and raise final weights in broilers by 7%. Additionally, very recent research has confirmed that broilers can have performance-enhancing benefits with enhanced body weight gain and feed intake of up to 6.6% and 6.9%, respectively. According to certain studies [He *et al.*, 2010; Zhang and Shao (1995); Adu*et al.*, 2011], broiler body weight increase has improved when REE supplements are added to the diet. In contrast to previous investigations, Xie and Wang (1998) discovered that high amounts of REE in the diet (300 mg/kg) had a detrimental impact on growth rate and feed conversion ratio. Agbede*et al.* (2011) and Schuller *et al.* (2002) demonstrated that lanthanum and REE, respectively, had no influence on production metrics. According to He *et al.* (2010), broiler performance was shown to be enhanced by REE-citrate; nevertheless, the exact mechanism by which REE might enhance animal performance remains unclear. Conversely, it has been suggested that REE may stimulate the release of gastrointestinal fluids (Ou *et al.*, 2000). According to Xu *et al.* (2004), lanthanum caused mice's stomachs to secrete more gastric acid.According to Pagano *et al.* (2015), Ce and La are two REEs that are often utilized as feed supplements for pigs and poultry, either in organic or inorganic form. In comparison to the use of inorganic REEs (e.g., REE-enriched yeast (RY) and REE-citrate), the addition of organic REEs (e.g., REE-enriched yeast (RY) and REE-citrate) to non-ruminant diets significantly increased the serum concentration of 3,5,3′ triiodothyronine, nutrient digestibility, and growth performance (Cai *et al.*, 2018; Forster *et al.*, 2008).

Rare earths have been shown to improve animal performance in certain studies, while in others, these benefits were either hardly noticeable or not noted at all. The degree to which rare earths improve performance can be attributed to a variety of factors, including the chemical used, concentration, and combination of rare earths used in the feeding trials. It is now unable to make a firm determination on the ideal composition. Nevertheless, a dose-dependency was noted in many experiments, and using a combination of rare earths rather than only lanthanum produced superior results. Furthermore, it appears that organic rare earth compounds affect animal performance more than inorganic ones do. This is likely due to distinct chemical properties that cause differences in absorption as well as bioavailability. In general, animals excrete more than 95% of the rare earths they are given orally, meaning that relatively little of them are absorbed. Oral toxicity of rare earths is relatively low, similar to regular table salt, based on minute gastrointestinal absorption. The range of LD50 values observed in several animal tests was 830 mg/kg to 10 g/kg body weight. Low oral toxicity and the safe use of rare earth feed additives for animals are further supported by the fact that no adverse effects on the health of the animals were noted in any of the feeding studies that were conducted. Furthermore, no impacts on the quality of the meat or carcass were noted. Similarly, organ samples showed very low quantities of rare earth elements, either the same or even lower than in control animals. This is explained by the fact that rare earth elements are found everywhere, even in plants and soil. They therefore show up in animal and human tissue as well as commercial diets. It has also been demonstrated that the levels of rare earth elements in typical vegetable diets remain greater than those in meat from animals given extra rare earths. As a result, it is also thought that adding rare earths to feed is safe for people. Furthermore, using rare earth elements in agriculture shouldn't harm the ecosystem, as far as we now know. Reducing environmental impacts from animal waste may actually help with the effective use of natural resources, as rare earths have the ability to improve feed conversion. As a result, rare earths are compliant with EU legislation on feed additive registration in terms of animal, human, and environmental safety. There are a few theories as to why rare earths have performance-enhancing properties, even if the mechanism is not fully known. Current research suggests that rare earths may operate locally in the gastrointestinal system, affecting nutrient intake, digestion, and utilization in addition to the bacterial microflora. Likewise, positive effects could potentially be influenced by anti-oxidative and anti-inflammatory properties. Actions on the intermediate metabolism that have an impact on immune system function, growth- and digestibility-related hormones and enzymes, or cellular processes have also been taken into consideration. It's also feasible that rare earths are not yet recognized as necessary components.

Research has shown that supplementing with cerium oxide in the diet dramatically reduced the levels of serum malondialdehyde (MDA) and the activity of superoxide dismutase (SOD) in egg yolks (Bolukbasi *et al*., 2016). According to Kawagoe *et al*. (2005), adding cerulean to rats' diets significantly decreased their plasma SOD activity, but had no effect on their plasma lipoperoxide (LPO) concentration. Furthermore, Redling (2006) proposed that dietary REEs' immunostimulant action may enhance the animal's overall health. The effects of feeding lanthanum oxide levels (0, 100, 200, 300, or 400 mg/kg) on laying performance, egg quality, yolk fatty acid content, egg lipid peroxidation, and some blood serum parameters of laying hens were studied by Durmus and Bolukbasi (2015).

Residual Impacts

It has been proposed that decreased gastrointestinal absorption of REEs in broiler chickens and piglets accounts for the low residual concentrations of Ce and La in the muscles and hepatic tissues (He et al., 2010; He et al., 2001).

Following product analysis, the safety of REE feed additives was tested on two million animals by the state technical inspection departments (IMSTID) in Inner Mongolia.The conclusion was that neither people nor animals could be poisoned by REEs or their additions (Rosewell, 1995). Consistently, Ming et al. (1995) concluded that the quality of animal feedstuffs and carcasses was unaffected by REE supplementation. Researchers Xie and Wang (1998) and Liu (2005) conducted additional trials in which they demonstrated that pigs supplemented with REEs did not significantly change slaughter indexes such as body length, carcass weight and thickness, back fat, eye muscle area, meat color and marbling, pH value, rate of lean meat, water holding, water loss, and cooked meat compared to control one. REEs have a strong affinity for bone, as evidenced by their high concentration in pig bone, as described by Ming et al. (1995). Furthermore, it has been observed that supplementing chickens with REEs led to the rabid removal of REEs from hepatic tissue as well as the preservation of meat quality; no significant accumulation of REEs was found in the chickens' muscle or liver (Xie and Wang, 1998). According to Zhou (1994), REE residues in meat and liver tissues of meat breed ducks ranged from 0.1 to 0.2 mg/kg, but only minimal levels were found in the eggs. According to Shi et al. (1990), REEs were found in fish, pigs, and chickens at low safe quantities. The largest concentrations were found in the bone, gill, and fin of the animals, although this buildup was quickly depilated. These data suggest that the use of REEs as feed additives at low concentrations appears to be safe for both people and animals. Based on these premises, feeding additives containing REEs to farm animals was deemed safe and appropriate for the most part.

Conclusion

Rare earth elements in the Earth's crust are estimated to have an average content of 130 to 240 mg/g, which is significantly higher than other metals have a positive impact on growth performance, nutrient utilization, antioxidant capacity, and egg production in poultry without any negative impact on birds' performance.

18

Commercial Guar Meal (CGM) An Alternate Protein Source in Poultry Feeding

[1]M. Hanumanth Rao, [2]Gurram Srinivas, [3]Swathi Bora and [4]Sushmasri Kandanulu

[1]Livestock Research Station, Mamnoor, Warangal, Telangana
[2]Poultry Research Station
[3]Veterinary Pathology
[4]ICAR -DPR
P.V. Narsimha Rao Telangana Veterinary University, Rajendranagar
Hyderabad, Telangana State

The profitability of poultry farming primarily depends on reduction in feed cost, which can be achieved by utilizing optimum concentrations of energy and crude protein (CP) from economically viable and nutritionally balanced feed ingredients. Soya bean meal (SBM) is conventionally used as a source of protein in poultry diet. However, the shortage and escalating cost of this prime protein source makes poultry farming uneconomical in many developing countries. Continuous efforts are, therefore, is on in search of viable alternate protein feed ingredients for SBM. Guar (*Cyamopsis tetragonoloba*) is a drought tolerant legume primarily cultivated for culinary preparations. Guar seeds are extracted for guar gum, which has a wide range of applications in pharmaceuticals, oil well drilling, ore floatation and paper making industries. To produce gum (galactomannan) guar seeds are split, which yields protein rich germ fraction and low protein husk fraction as by- products (Conner, 2002). Guar meal (GM) is a combination of these two fractions, which contains similar amount of CP and less expensive than SBM (Rama Rao *et al.*, 2014).

Production Status and Nutrient Composition of Guar in India

Guar seed production in India fluctuates from year to year based on rainfall pattern, area of cultivation and yield (Multi Commodity Exchange of India Ltd., 2009). Rajasthan wholly retains the credit for India's position producing 70% of the production followed by Gujarat, Haryana and Punjab. The major markets for guar seed are Jodhpur, Bikaner, Ganganagar, Jaipur, Alwar etc. The country exports over 1,17,000 tons of guar by-products, which is comprised of 33000 tons of refined split guar gum and 84000 tons of treated and pulverized guar gum. However SA is the biggest consumer of guar gum with an annual consumption of 45,000 tonnes which represents 25% of world trade.

Table 1: Production status of guar in India

Year	Production (lakh tonnes)
2011 – 12	22.18
2012 – 13	24.61
2013- 14	27.15

Table 2: Nutrient composition of GM, GNC and SBM.

Nutrient	GM	GNC	SBM
ME, kcal/kg	1821	2103	2205
CP, %	37.1	38.8	44.9
Lysine, %	2.58	1.61	2.66
Methionine, %	0.39	0.44	0.62
Arginine, %	5.90	4.79	3.11
Calcium, %	0.41	0.17	0.29
Non phytin phosphorus, %	0.15	0.18	0.26

Source: Reddy and Bhosale, 2001.

Feeding Aspects of Guar Meal

The bitter taste and presence of anti-nutritional factors limit the use of GM in poultry feeds. Trypsin inhibitors inhibit the proteolytic activity of trypsin and chymotrypsin. Trypsin inhibitor activity in raw GM contributes towards decrease growth performance of poultry. Furthermore, many researchers reported that diets containing raw GM results in reduced bodyweight, feed consumption and feed efficiency in poultry. This poor performance of poultry birds might be attributed to increased pancreatic secretions and decreased protease activity.

Trypsin inhibitor activity can be overcome by heat treatment or by supplementation of essential amino acids such as methionine, and can be destroyed by extrusion processing. Couch *et al.* (1967) reported approximately 80% reduction in trypsin inhibitor activity by heating GM for 60 minutes.

Furthermore observed the harmful effects of trypsin inhibitor which can be alleviated by heating GM up to 110ºC for 1 hour with 15 minutes of super heated steam. However while studying the harmful effects of GM feeding, many researchers found that trypsin inhibitors were not the primary factors for deleterious effects of GM to poultry. Furthermore, heating and steam pelleting diets having GM had no effect on the performance of broiler chicks (Verma and McNab,1982).Growth suppressing effects in animals by anti-nutritional factors present in GM, notably antitrypsin inhibitors, are less certain than others, because during gum extraction processes guar seeds are passed through a temperature range of 93.3- 105ºC (Lee *et al*., 2004).

Guar gum (galactomannan polysaccharide) is sticky in nature. Germ and hull fractions of GM contain variable quantity of residual gum that is remnant of gum extraction from the guar seeds. Gum residues make intestinal material more viscous, resulting in lowered nutrient uptake by the gastrointestinal tract (GIT) and reduced nutrient availability.

Although NSPs (galactomannan in GM) are poorly digested by monogastric animals and linked with decreased nutrient utilization, dietary NSPs can affect intestinal ecosystem by provision of fermentable substrates which encourages the growth of beneficial bacterial species and prevents establishment and colonization by pathogenic bacteria in the epithelial tissues within the GIT. Furthermore, undigested or partially digested NSPs at the distal end of GI tract can be a nutrient source of short chain fatty acids(SCFAs) which are of energetic importance to the host animals, and in poultry are readily absorbed by the colonic mucosa. Residual gum present in GM contains β-1-4 glycosidic linkages which cannot be digested by animals, but are well fermented by microbes in the GIT and SCFA production. This causes decreasing luminalP^H and thus inhibits the growth and proliferation of pathogens in GI tract. Additionally gum residues have been reported to improve macrophage activity.

Alleviation of Deleterious Factors

Orga *et al.* (1962) noticed that heating or steaming of GM improved its nutritional value slightly while Phillips (1963) claimed to have detoxified the GM markedly by heat treatment. Bakshi *et al.* (1964) reported that chicks utilized heated or autoclaved GM better than raw one. Vohra and Kratzer (1964) reported that chicks utilized heated or autoclaved GM by treating it with the slurry containing sprouted guar bean and it was found that such combination was more toxic than GM alone. However, diets containing 20 % toasted or autoclaved GM along with 0.1 or 0.2 % cellulose produced a marked improvement in the growth of chicks. Nagpal *et al. (*1971) found that neither autoclaving nor addition of DL-methionine and L-lysine significantly improved the protein value of GM. Brahma *et al*. (1979) reported that addition of DL-methionine to TGM containing diet improved BWG, FCR and protein efficiency ratio. Verma and Mc Nab, (1984) did not show any improvement in the performance of broilers by toasting GM, steam pelleting or supplementation with 5 g methionine per kg diet. GM cooked in the presence of moisture improves its feeding value and that an effective enzyme supplementation should be used when GM more than 10% or more is used (Patel and McGinnis, 1985). Trypsin inhibitor can be destroyed by cooking the raw GM for a period 1h at a temperature of 110ºC with super heated steam for a period of 15 minutes after the cooker attains a temperature of 110ºC (Ramamani,1986).

Autoclaving the raw GM resulted in considerable destruction of haemagglutinin (84%) and trypsin inhibitor (84 %) without much changing the saponin (6.1 %) and phytate (7.5 %) contents. Acidified water leaching of autoclaved meal decreased the concentrations of saponin to 2.1 %, phytate 3.9 % and polyphenols 0.76 %. Extracting the meal with aqueous alcohols lowered the concentration of free polyphenols to 0.17-0.27%, haemagglutinin to nil and phytate to 3.5 % besides complete leaching out of saponins. Raw GM supported only 88% of growth of control while acid leached autoclaved GM supported 96% of growth of control. No gross pathological symptoms were observed in chicks fed processed GM (Rajput *et al*., 1998). As the incriminating factor present in raw GM is heat sensitive, it is presumed that heat treatment may improve the nutritional value of GM and it can be used in poultry rations at higher levels.

Conclusions

From the research studies conducted and the results obtained the following conclusions can be drawn

1. Heat processed guar meal could be a valuable alternative to soya bean meal as it is a protein rich feed stuff possessing nearly 48% CP on DMB, considerable amount of all essential amino acids, calcium (0.46%), phosphorus ((0.60%) and a moderate source of energy (2453 Kcal/Kg)
2. Heat processed guar meal can be included up to 10% in broiler rations containing Maize-soya bean with effecting BWG, FI, FCR, nutrient utilization and carcass traits
3. Heat processed guar meal can be included up to 18% in White Leghorn layer rations with effecting Performance, Egg quality and Serum biochemical variables

19

Role of Poultry Nutrition in Fertility and Hatchability

V.D. Lonkar

Department of Poultry Science, KNP College of Veterinary Science Shirwal, Dist. Satara. 412 801, Maharashtra Animal & Fishery Sciences University, Nagpur , Maharashtra India

Laying and broiler breeding are the backbone of the poultry industry. Fertility and hatchability are the two most important reproductive traits of breeder birds that highly influence the supply of quality day-old commercial chicks and growth of poultry industry. Fertility and hatchability are parameters of economic viability (King'Ori, 2011; Malik *et al.,* 2015) and interrelated heritable traits that vary among breeds, variety and individuals in a breed or variety. Fertility refers to the average percentage of eggs that were fertilized and hatchability refers to the proportion of chicks hatched from the total number of eggs set for incubation (hatchability on the basis of total egg set), and based on the total number of fertile eggs (hatchability on the basis of fertile eggs set) (Wolc *et al.,* 2019). Both the male and female breeder birds take part in the production of fertile eggs. After mating the sperm from the male bird is released into the female reproductive tract which reaches upto the infundibulum of the female oviduct where the sperm unite with ovum to produce zygote which results in fertile egg. Fertile egg contains blastoderm at oviposition. Egg cannot hatch if not fertile (Ogbu and Oguike, 2019). The fertility and hatchability are multifactorial influenced reproductive traits that includes both genetic and non-genetic factors (King'Ori, 2011 and Ogbu and Oguike, 2019). Heritability estimates for fertility and hatchability are very low in chicken that range from 0.06 to 0.13 (Saap *et. al.,* 2004). This indicate that the non-genetic factors like nutrition have higher influence on these two traits.

Why Nutrition of the Breeder Flock is Important?

Maintenance of fertility of modern broiler breeders during the breeding period is one of the biggest challenges faced by poultry breeders. The nutrients in the feed are essential for breeding birds to invest some nutrients in the egg. Balanced nutrients in diet prevent excessive weight gain, which is a a major cause of poor-quality ejaculate, testicular regression in males and ovulation and early ovarian regression in females (Brillard, 2007). Diet affects reproduction in the chicken in three ways: It affects the quantity and fertilizing capacity of the sperm produced by the males and thereby affects the number of fertilized eggs, production and composition of eggs and thus, in turn, hatchability of fertile eggs. The nutrients profile of egg changes with the maternal diet (An *et al.,* 2010; Nonis and Gous, 2013) and thereby creates differences in the nutritional status of progeny (Ajuyah *et al.,* 2003). Both maternal and paternal nutrition plays an important role to maximize the number of eggs per breeder bird, to obtain high hatchability with a high fertility rate, to maximize the number of good quality chicks per breeder bird, to minimize mortality and culling rate, and to prevent deficiency diseases in the chicks. Bodyweight profile and frame size in male and female and; fleshing and carcass conformation of males are influenced by the nutrient composition of breeder diet and thereby influences the flock uniformity (Zuidhof *et al.,* 2017). Equitable feed allocation and stable metabolic rates are likely to increase flock uniformity and reproductive efficiency.

During chick and growing stage, dietary nutrients determine the future performance and focus on the skeletal, intestinal, cardiovascular, and immune systems development with flock uniformity. Pre-breeder and peak production feeding is crucial for breeder females to achieve sexual maturation, egg production, maximum number of fertile hatching eggs with emphasis on chick quality during the initial phase and hatchability during the late production. Specific feeding strategies should be adopted to avoid a drop in production and hatchability during the post-peak production phase. For male breeder birds separate feeding, feeding to improve semen quality and fertility has to be adopted (Chang *et al.,* 2016). Nutritional factors greatly modulate aging effect on reproductive organs, semen quality and fertility of poultry males.

During the rearing period, males can be fed the same diets as females. However, separate control of male feeding levels during the reproductive period using sex-separate feeding systems is essential. Separate sex feeding especially males control body weight and improve uniformity. The use of a single feed for both sexes is usually practiced during period of laying. However, specific male diet during this time found to be beneficial for maintenance of reproductive function (Moyle *et al.,* 2011).

Effect of Energy and Protein on Fertility and Hatchability

Energy is the first limiting "nutrient" for breeder birds. Therefore, breeder bird should be fed with appropriate energy during both rear and lay to fulfil maintenance requirements, support growth, daily egg production, and egg size (Silva, 2014). Feeding of low protein and medium to high energy in breeder diets during rearing and laying period had a positive impact on egg production, egg size, breeder fertility, hatchability, embryonic livability and on offspring performance (Chang *et al.*, 2016). Excess energy is stored as fat that increases body weight and heavier body weight reduces both hatchability and fertility. In other hands, decreased energy intake has been shown to negatively affect the sperm concentration and total live sperm (Bramwell *et al.*, 1996).

Dietary protein has strongest effect on breeder males. Consistent improvement in fertility was observed when roosters were fed with specific male diet compared with the female diet. Feeding of 6.9% protein in layer males had higher fertility than 16.9% protein fed males (Arscot and Parker, 1963). The number of broiler breeders were increased when fed with 9 % dietary protein compared to 12 and 15% protein fed broiler breeders (Wilson *et al.*, 1987) while 12% protein fed male breeders had higher sperm concentration compared to 16% protein (Hocking and Bernard, 1997). Longer fertile period in broiler breeders was achieved by CP of 12.5% (Tyler and Bekker, 2012). The protein levels of 11.7 to 12.6% for male broiler breeders was recommended by Rostagno *et al.* (2011).

Silveira *et al.* (2014) studied the specific-male diet on fertility and hatchability. The diet formulated for females contained average 2830 kcal ME/kg and 15% CP, while diet specifically formulated for male broiler breeders contained 2750 kcal ME/kg and 13.5% CP. They reported that specific breeder male diet has beneficial effects on body weight and egg hatchability and fertility. Thus, specific male breeder diet increases the number of chicks hatched.

Reddy and Rama Rao (2001) suggested 15% CP and 2850 kcal/kg ME for male egg type breeders. Shanmugam *et al.* (2016) that the reduced dietary CP (16% to 8.97%) with constant ME level (2950kcal/kg) had no effect on semen and fertility parameters in layer breeder males (Dahlem Red) but levels of protein and energy combinations had influence on percent abnormal sperm, fertility and hatchability in layer breeder males. When both CP and ME was reduced (2360kcal/kg ME, 9 % CP), the percent abnormal sperm was significantly ($P<0.05$) lowered. The average fertility was significantly ($P<0.05$) higher in the High energy low protein diet (2950kcal/kg ME, 8.97% CP) diet and the average hatchability was lower in the low energy low protein (2360kcal/kg ME, 9 % CP) diet. It seems that the dietary protein level can be reduced up to 9% level without affecting the reproductive efficiency of the layer breeder males but in practice, layer breeder males are provided diet having 13%-15% CP.

Effect of Fat type / Oil Sources on Fertility and Hatchability

Dietary fatty acids have effect on sperm quality, hen's egg fatty acid content and chick embryonic development. Fats in the egg yolk are the main energy source for the developing chick embryo (Aydin & Cook, 2009). Lipid peroxidation affect sperm cells. Due to specific proportions of sperm fatty acids, dietary lipid sources affect sperm composition and functionality (Bongalhardo *et al.*, 2009).

Polyunsaturated fatty acids (PUFAs) play significant roles in metabolism, endocrine function, plasma membrane fluidity in sperm and functions related to fertilization events (Masoudi *et al.*, 2016). In avian species, the percentage of n-6 polyunsaturated fatty acids (n-6 PUFAs) is found to be higher in spermatozoa and seminal plasma (Surai *et al.*, 2001; Cerolini *et al., 2003*). This indicating that n-6 PUFAs play important roles in the formation and characteristics of sperm, and thus fertility. However, PUFAs are strongly susceptible to lipid peroxidation that induces the production of ROS that interfere with damage to sperm function (Surai *et al.*, 2001; Cerolini *et al.*, 2000; Emamverdi *et al.*, 2015). Especially in the aged rooster, unprotected PUFAs supplementation cause sperm function loss and the endocrine system (Cerolini *et al.*, 2005). Lipids rich in n-3 PUFAs increased the fertility in cockerels fed a diet containing 2% menhaden oil, leading to increased numbers of fertilized eggs when hens were artificially inseminated once in three weeks (Hudson and Wilson, 2003). Fish oil enhances fatty acid oxidation by promoting activity of mitochondria and beta oxidation in birds fed a diet containing fish oil. This could affect the energy production, which may explain why dietary fish oil enhances the forward progressive motility (Poureslami *et al.*, 2010). Inclusion of 4% fish oil increased fertility compared with a basal diet containing corn oil. Inclusion of 6% linseed oil increased fertility in Cobb breeders (Kelso *et al.*, 1997) while 2% linseed oil increased fertility and sperm content of EPA and DHA in Ross roosters (Zanussi *et al.*, 2019). The enhanced fertility of roosters induced by diets containing linseed oil may be attributed to increased sperm motility due to improved energy production by the activation of beta oxidation (Ferrini *et al.*, 2010). Qi *et al.* (2019) also found that, 2% linseed oil enhanced semen volume, sperm viability, motility, and total sperm count by enhancing testosterone synthesis via upregulation of the mRNA expression levels of rate-limiting enzymes involved in steroidogenesis (Qi *et al.*, 2019). Olubowale *et al.* (2014) reported that the inclusion of either combination of 1.5% fish oil plus 1.5% linseed oil or 3% High Oleic Acid sunflower oil maiantain sperm motility, at the end of the production cycle in breeder layer hens during 69-77 weeks of age. Recently, Saber and Kutlu (2020) reported that the dietary omega-3 and omega-6 FA did not affect ($p<0.05$) number of fertile eggs, embryonic mortality in early and mid stage, and fertility rate. However, the inclusion of omega-3 and omega-6 fatty acids sources in breeder diets had a significant ($p<0.05$) effect on late-stage embryo mortality, hatchability of fertile eggs and total hatchability. Asl *et al.* (2018) studied the effect of n-3: n-6 FA ratios (0.09, 0.16, and 0.23) based on the inclusion of three oil sources (1% canola oil plus1% fish oil, and 2% fish oil) in aged Ross broiler breeders (45 week-old) and reported that fertility was affected by the different ratios of n-3: n-6 (*0.16 and 0.23*) but hatchability was unaffected.

The supplementation of different oil sources containing omega-3 and omega-6 fatty acids seems to be beneficial in improving fertility and hatchability of breeder flocks.

Effect of Antioxidants on Fertility and Hatchability

Vitamin E and Se are the potent antioxidants being used in poultry diet. Vitamin E, carotenoids and Se can be transferred from the diet to the egg and consequently to the developing embryo (Surai, 2002). Chance *et al.* (1979) reported that about 2 x10^{10} molecules of reactive oxygen species (ROS) are generated per day in a cell and their rate increases in stress condition. The free radicals are formed as a natural consequence of the body's normal metabolic activity and as part of the immune system's strategy. The antioxidants are present naturally in living organisms and they are the major factor that enables their survival in an oxygen-rich environment termed as antioxidant system (Surai, 2002). These ROS protects the cell from damage. These includes vitamins E, Vitamin A, carotenoids etc. (natural fat-soluble antioxidants), ascorbic acid, uric acid, taurine, etc. (water-soluble antioxidants); antioxidant enzymes like glutathione peroxidase (GSH-Px), catalase (CAT) and superoxide dismutase (SOD); thiol redox system consisting of the glutathione system (Surai, 2002). Presence of extremely high proportions of long–chain PUFA in the phospholipid fraction of spermatozoa is the most important feature of lipid composition of avian semen. This high PUFA proportion is required to maintain fluidity and flexibility which are the specific membrane properties. Due to the presence of lipids, spermatozoa became very susceptible to lipid peroxidation. Therefore, antioxidants are most important to maintain semen quality.

The storage of spermatozoa within an oviducal sperm storage tubule, enables the hen to produce fertile eggs during the 'fertile period' of 1–6 weeks, depending on the species. Thus, avian spermatozoa might be expected to have systems which maintain stability throughout this period. It has been shown that during sperm storage, lipid peroxidation is associated with a significant decrease in PUFA concentration in spermatozoa.

Selenium (Se) as a part of various selenoproteins can help maintain antioxidant defences preventing damages to tissues. Se supplementation is known to affect the antioxidant defences of chicken semen (Surai *et al.*, 1998). Edens (2002) reported only 57.9% normal spermatozoa when cockerels were fed on a basal diet containing 0.28 ppm Se without additional dietary supplementation. He found bent midpiece (18.7%) and corkscrew head (15.4%) sperm abnormalities. However, percentage of normal spermatozoa increased to 89.4% and abnormalities in the form of bent midpiece and corkscrew head were decreased down to 6.2 and 1.8% respectively, when this diet was supplemented with an additional 0.2 ppm Se in the form of selenite. The further improvement in semen quality was observed by inclusion of same amount of organic Se (abnormalities decreased down to 0.7 and 0.2% and the percentage of normal spermatozoa increased up to 98.7%). Surai (2006) recommended 0.2–0.3 ppm of selenium in organic form for supplementation in breeders. The organic Se being much more effective in comparison to selenite. Organic selenium can also improve fertility and, more importantly, increase the duration of fertility (Agate *et al.*, 2000). Se supplementation in the organic form is shown to positively affect hatchability (Renema, 2003). Selenium from the albumen is transferred to embryo during first two weeks of the embryo development, while Se from egg yolk is delivered to theembryo during last week of incubation (Surai, 2006).

Increased vitamin E concentration (Surai *et al.*, 1999) and carotenoid concentration (Surai *et al.*, 2003) in the chicken embryonic tissues were associated with decreased tissue susceptibility to lipid peroxidation. Vitamin E is one of the main sperm antioxidants which was detected abundantly in sperm membrane (Surai *et al.*, 2000), and it protects sperm cells from oxidative damage (Rooke *et al.*, 2001). Dietary supplementation of Vit E along with lipid sources prevented the occurrence or progression of lipid peroxidation of sperm (Asl *et al.*, 2018). Combination of vitamin E (200 mg/kg) and organic Se (0.3 mg/kg) in the cockerel's diet enhanced spermatozoa count and motility, and reduced percentage of dead spermatozoa (Ebeid, 2012).

Effect of Trace Minerals on Fertility and Hatchability

Trace minerals such as iron, manganese (Mn), zinc (Zn), copper (Cu), and selenium (Se) play many significant roles as enzyme cofactors and as constituents of metalloenzymes. The antioxidant glutathione peroxidase (GSH-Px), containing selenium (Se) in its activity center, which can improve GSH-Px catalytic activity directly, plays a crucial role in protecting sperm from oxidative damage (Moslemi & Tavanbakhsh, 2011). Zinc plays a role in the stabilization of the sperm membrane, preventing its degradation (Taniguchi *et al.,* 2007). Zinc is a crucial component of antioxidant enzymes [metallothioneins (MT) and copper-zinc superoxide dismutase (CuZnSOD)] in avian semen, which could protect the spermatozoal membrane and increase spermatozoal viability. Copper also plays important role in reproduction. Prostaglandin E2 (PGE2) can regulate the synthesis of LH through copper, increasing LH serum levels, thereby inducing testosterone secretion to promote the differentiation and maturation of sperm cells (Sakumoto *et al.,* 2014). Manganese trace element present in all tissues and it is fundamental for the normal metabolism of amino acid, lipid, protein, and carbohydrate (Zhu & Richards, 2017). Manganese is usually supplemented in broiler breeder feeds as part of the micro-mineral premix, frequently as a sulfate salt, but sometimes incorporated in a diversity of organic minerals.

Zinc deficiency in poultry breeder birds led to lower semen quality (reducing around 10% sperm motility) and egg production (lowering 3–10 g/day/bird egg mass) as well as poor offspring development and growth performance (increasing 9–10% weak chick ratio and 10% mortality of progeny) (Huang *et al.,* 2019). Zinc is an essential trace mineral in breeder hen diets, and a 50-mg Zn/kg diet is recommended to maintain the optimum productive performance by the National Research Council. Adding Zn in a pure form used as an efficient tool for improving the reproductive performance of poultry breeders. Amen *et al.* (2011) evaluated the effect of Zn (0, 50, 100 mg/kg diet on fertility traits and sperm-egg penetration of Cobb-500 broiler breeders (45week age). Hens were artificially inseminated with semen during 51, 54, 57, 60, and 66 weeks of age for fertility traits study and they found that adding Zn in the diet significantly increased fertility, hatchability of total egg set, hatchability of fertile eggs. The sperm-egg penetration was also increased significantly during 54, 58, 62, and 66 weeks. Sperm penetration of ovum Inner Perivitelline Layer (IPVL) is positively correlated with fertility. A greater number of sperm penetration holes in the IPVL are indicative of successful insemination and can be positively associated with optimum filling of the sperm storage tubules

(SST) in the uterovaginal region of the oviduct (Fairchild, 2001). Amen *et al.* (2011) suggested that 100 mg Zn/kg in the diet is required to obtain optimal fertility, hatchability, and sperm-egg penetration traits in broiler breeder chicken. Sahin and Tasdemir (2017) reported that 60 mg/kg organic-based zinc (Zn-RedoxMin) supplementation instead of inorganic sources (ZnSO4, ZnO, and ZnC12) to breeder diets improved their chick quality. Stanley *et al.*, 2012 reported that early and late embryonic mortality was significantly ($P<0.05$) lower in eggs from hens provided diets containing Se+Zn. Zhu *et al.* (2015) supplementing 120 ppm Mn on a deficient diet (14.3 ppm Mn in a corn-soybean meal diet) have observed improvements in hatchability of eggs 359 from broiler breeder hens (88.8 to 95.1%). Taschetto *et al.* (2017) reported that the average dietary Fe requirement for broiler breeder's hen estimated to be about 100 ppm total.

Recommendation for using organic-based (chelated) trace minerals, containing a central metal atom (acceptor of electrons) together with ligands *(i.e.*, proteins, amino acids, carbohydrates, or lipids), at relatively low levels in poultry diets has become widespread (Swinkels *et al.*, 1994). Organic trace minerals (OTM) present a better rate of absorption and utilization, good chemical stability, higher biological potency, and delay the antagonism among different minerals than inorganic and simple organic trace minerals (Spears, 1996). Organic trace minerals have been increasingly used in poultry feeds due to their higher bioavailability, that is, their higher utilization capacity compared with inorganic trace minerals. Due to their high bioavailability, OTM in broiler diets reduce trace mineral excretion in the environment (Bao *et al.*, 2007).

Sun *et al.* (2012) reported that adding an organic form of Zn, Mn, and Se (Mintrex) instead of an inorganic form of these microelements in broiler breeders diet protected breeders from lipid peroxidation, increase their retention in the egg, and had a positive effect on growth performance of their offspring. Saber *et al.* (2020) investigated the effects of dietary inorganic and/or organic-based trace mineral premix (Mn, Fe, Zn, Cu, Se, Co, and I) in full or half doses in broiler breeder (36 week-old) diet and showed that diets containing full (100%) or half (50%) doses of organic and/or inorganic minerals in broiler breeder hens diet had a significant effect on fertility rate ($P<0.05$). They concluded that replacing inorganic-based trace mineral premix with half or full dose of organic-based trace mineral premix in the broiler breeder hens' diet could improve hatching performance, growth, and carcass performances of their progenies. Feeding organic trace minerals premix (OTM) to male broilers breeders improves ($p<0.05$) semen quality from 31 to 35 weeks, which may be attributed to their better testicular development and higher expression of enzymes (mRNA expression of the genes 3-beta dehydrogenase 2 and cytochrome P450 17A1) related to testosterone synthesis at 45 weeks (Shan *et al.*, 2017). Organic trace minerals had a positive impact on the growth of closed-packed spermatogonia and Leydig cells. Du *et al.* (1996) and Mondal *et al.* (2007) that inorganic trace element does not fulfil trace element requirements of modern poultry due to their less bioavailability and negative interaction. Araujo *et al.*, (2019) reported that the organic trace mineral (OTM) supplementation improved Cobb-500 broiler breeder hens' performance in terms of higher egg production and better eggshell quality compared with that fed ITM but the Egg fertility and hatchability were not influenced.

Effect of Vitamins on Fertility and Hatchability

Vitamins represents less than 1 % of cost of poultry feed but important for metabolic functions in poultry. Breeder birds' diets are supplemented with higher vitamin levels as compared to commercial poultry diets. Vitamin A deficiency causes decreased in performance, infertility leads to impaired reproduction (Clagett-Dame and DeLuca, 2002). Today, broiler breeding companies recommend 10,000 IU/kg vitamin as the requirement level of broilers or broiler breeders (Ross broiler breeder nutrition specification 2007). Higher levels of vitamin A (210,000 to 410,000 IU/kg) decreased egg production, size, and hatchability in laying hens (March et al., 1972). However, Yuan *et al.* (2014) reported that vitamin A levels up to and including 35,000 IU/kg did not affect reproductive performance. Broiler breeders supplemented more than 35,000 IU Vitamin A /kg diet has been shown to impair liver function, reproductive performance, and immune response. Vitamin A supplementation ranging between 5,000 IU/kg to 35,000 IU/kg did not affect hatchability in breeders.

Vitamin E is supplemented in male breeder diet to improve reproductive status. Studies by Breque *et al.* (2003) indicate a positive effect of dietary vitamin E on the antioxidant status of sperm storage sites in hens. In avian species, sperm proportion found at sperm storage tubule of utero-vaginal junction significantly correlate with the sperms found at perivitelline layer of eggs (Brillard, 1993; Brillard and Bakst, 1990). Lin *et al.* (2005) found that that the maximum duration of fertility was improved by supplementing 160 mg/kg vitamin E at 49 weeks of age in Taiwan native chicken. Khan *et al.* (2013) found that additional vitamin E and C or their combination was the most potent nutrient treatment for improving the semen quality. Supplementation of vitamin E (100 IU/kg) and C (500 IU/kg) had significantly higher semen volume compared to control. Vitamin E (100 IU/kg) supplemented birds had higher sperm motility and vitamin C (500 IU/kg) supplemented group had lower dead spermatozoa percentage compared to control. They also found that the seminal plasma total antioxidant capacity was higher in the vitamin E group. The dietary increase in the vitamin E inside semen was demonstrated to determine a significant decrease in the lipid peroxidation susceptibility (Lin *et al.,* 2005). Absence of vitamin E in basal diet decrease fertility and it was restored after supplementation Biswas *et al.* (2007). Inclusion of vitamin E in cockerels diet significantly decreased the abnormal and dead spermatozoa proportion and improved fertility was observed by Biswas *et al.* (2009). Decrease in fertility with advanced age was also linked with lower testicular vitamin E levels which was restored gain by supplementing vitamin E (Surai *et al.,* 2000). Thus, dietary vitamin E significantly supports reproductive functions in avian species.

Min *et al.* (2016) observed that supplemental dietary vitamin C and vitamin E in combination enhanced serum testosterone and sperm motility remarkably ($P<0.05$).

Single vitamins from Vitamin B group were deleted from the diet of breeding hens, and were then reintroduced 15 weeks later. Absence of B group vitamins for over three weeks period, individually, led to more than ten percent reduction in hatchability. After 15 weeks of feeding with deficient rations the missing vitamin was reintroduced. After 4 weeks of receiving the proper level of all vitamins, the breeders regained the standard levels of production and hatchability. Reduced production of hatching egg by start and end of laying period is related to the composition of egg and vitamin composition is pointed out as key factor (Lesson and Summers, 2005)

An inadequate quantity of biotin in breeders feed gives rise to a decrease in laying and hatchability with high mortality during the last week of incubation. When breeder feed contained biotin 165 µg/kg of biotin, the fertile eggs had a hatchability of 84%. When the dose of biotin was higher (440 µg/kg), hatchability reached 89%. (Robel, 1989). Biotin and riboflavin are vitamins with important characteristics due to the presence of the inhibitors avidin and ovo-flavoprotein in egg albumen, which affects their availability to the embryo. Deficiencies of these two vitamins are not uncommon, and may affect egg hatchability in just a few days after the hens are fed deficient diets (Leeson *et al.,* 1979). Folic acid is a critical vitamin for all animals during reproduction, and its requirement for hatchability is higher as compared to egg production (Taylor, 1947). Adequate levels of vitamins and minerals in breeder layer diets are important to support fertility, hatchability and normal embryo development, avoiding possible deficiencies that might cause death, malformation and other abnormalities like shortened legs and beak, clubbed down, perosis, edema, abnormal feathering, accelerated oxidative metabolism during late incubation.

Effect of Phytochemicals on Fertility of Males

Yan *et al.* (2017) determined the effects of turmeric on the semen quality in roosters. They found that 0.8 mg of turmeric by product/kg diet enhanced the sperm motility, thereby suggesting that the fertility could have been enhanced, although this was not tested. In addition, different levels of curcumin (10, 20, and 30 mg/rooster/d) were added to the diet of aged roosters (Kazemizadeh *et al.*, 2019). The authors found that the use of 30 mg of curcumin/rooster/d led to reductions in the abnormal sperm number, increases in live sperm, and decreased seminal lipid peroxidation. These findings were also accompanied by increases in the sperm membrane integrity, sperm motility, penetration, and fertility. Several studies have indicated that curcumin can enhance the antioxidant status in poultry (Zhang *et al.*, 2015; Ruan *et al.*, 2019) as well as increase the numbers of Leydig cells, spermatogonia cells, and the seminiferous tubule diameter, thereby enhancing the testicular weight and its function (Kazemizadeh *et al.*, 2018). These changes could explain the increases in the sperm membrane integrity and sperm concentration.

Ginger contains gingerol, gingerdiol, and gingerdione, which may promote the functioning of the antioxidant defense system. The antioxidant capacity was enhanced in chickens and laying hens when their diet was supplemented with ginger (Zhang *et al.*, 2009). These findings suggest that ginger might enhance the fertility of male poultry. Indeed, adding 15 g of ginger root powder/kg diet increased the fertility of aged Cobb male breeders (Akhlaghi *et al.*, 2014). Ginger increased sperm production because of improved testes growth by enhancing development of the seminiferous tubules and germ cells and semen quality by suppressing the oxidative damage induced in the testes (Herve *et al.*, 2018).

Lycopene is an abundant carotenoid in tomatoes and red fruits, and it can neutralize free radicals and inhibit oxidative damage in cells. Drinking water containing lycopene (5.0 g/L) improved the fertility of roosters (Mangiagalli *et al.*, 2010). The semen quality characteristics also improved in roosters fed diets containing 15% dried tomato pomace, with an increase in the live sperm number and decrease in the number of defective sperm (Saemi *et al.*, 2012). Other carotenoids might also affect the fertility of male poultry. A diet containing 6.0 mg of canthaxanthin/kg increased the fertility (Rosa *et al.*, 2012) by improving the antioxidant status (Ren *et al.*, 2016). Supplementation with 5.0

g of rosemary leaf powder/kg diet increased the semen amount, concentration, and quality characteristics, including the live sperm number, forward motility, and sperm penetration (Borghei-Rad *et al.*, 2017), by increasing the diameter of the seminiferous tubules and the thickness of the germinal cell layer. Thus, increases in sperm biosynthesis occurred, as well as the enhanced production of GSH-Px and catalase to protect the testes and semen from oxidative damage (Turk *et al.*, 2016). Dietary supplementation with 0.25 mg of cinnamon bark oil/kg diet reduced lipid peroxidation, maintained the vitality of the testicular tissues, and increased the thickness of the germinal cell layer and sperm production (Turk *et al.*, 2015), but the effects on fertility were not evaluated. A diet containing 20% dried apple pomace increased the PUFA content in sperm and the total antioxidant capacity to reduce lipid peroxidation as well as improve the sperm fluidity and its forward movement to enhance sperm penetration and fertility (Akhlaghi *et al.*, 2014). Clearly, the concentrations of the active compounds present in different supplements will determine their effects. Table 1 summarizes the nutrients and feed additives that may enhance the fertility of male poultry.

Conclusions

Managing the modern breeder is an exhilarating challenge. Due to high reproductive potential of these birds, correct nutrition is of immense importance to achieve their full reproductive potential with respect to fertility and hatchability. Both the maternal and paternal nutritional factors influence fertility and hatchability of breeder poultry and allows to overcome low-fertility and hatchability problems, especially in aging breeder flocks, thereby obtaining beneficial impact on the poultry industry. Various nutritional factors like energy, protein, fats, amino acids and their metabolites, minerals, vitamins and phytochemicals significantly affect the fertility and hatchability. Specific male nutrition enhances the semen quality, protecting sperm against oxidative damage which help to optimize the sperm membrane functionality, sperm-egg penetration and thus fertility. Dietary CP can be reduced up to 9% in layer breeders and 13.5 % in broiler breeder diets without affecting fertility and hatchability (In practice, 14%-15% CP) - lower feed cost. Energy levels of 2950 kcal ME/kg diet in layer breeders and 2700-2750 kcal ME/kg diet in broiler breeders maintain best fertility and hatchability. Amino acids & their metabolite like L-threonine (0.12%), L-arginine (2.33g/kg diet), L-carnitine (125-150mg/kg diet) and D-aspartic acid (200 mg/kg BW) maintain best fertility in aged breeder males. Inclusion of n3 & n6 FUFA sources of oils like fish oil (2-5%) or linseed oil (2-6%) or combination of fish oil and Linseed oil (1.5% + 1.5%) or high oleic acid sunflower oil (3%) or flaxseed oil (2%) in feed improves fertility and hatchability. Addition of 50% inorganic + 50% organic trace minerals or 100% organic trace minerals containing Zn, Mn, Cu, Se, Fe, I in breeder diets improves semen quality as well as testosterone levels and testicular morphology. Dietary organic Se (0.2-0.4 mg/kg) or Zn (100mg/kg) or combination of Zn+Se helps to improves fertility and hatchability in breeder birds as well as reduce early and late embryonic mortality during incubation of hatching eggs, Vitamin A (35000 IU/kg), C (75 mg/kg), E (100mg/kg), Biotin (150-250µg/kg), Niacin (55mg/kg), B1 (2-2.5mg/kg), B2 (5-7mg/kg) maintain optimum fertility and hatchability. Phytochemicals like canthaxanthin (6 mg /kg diet), , Gingerol (15 g /kg diet), Gingerdiol (15 g /kg diet), Curcumin (30 mg /bird/day), and Lycopene (5.0 g/L water) having antioxidant properties improve fertility.

20

Indigenous Poultry A Sustainable Tool for Nutrition and Livelihood Security

***R.C. Kulkarni*[1] *and K. Sai Siva Kumar*[2]**

[1]*Department of Poultry Science, College of Veterinary and Animal Sciences Udgir, Maharashtra*
Maharashtra Animal and Fishery Sciences University, Udgir Maharashtra
[2]*Department of Poultry Science, ICAR-IVRI, Izatnagar, Bareilly Uttar Pradesh*

There has been a paradigm shift in the poultry sector regarding its structure and operations. Over five decades, backyard farming has transformed into a dynamic commercial agri-business. The poultry raised commercially is more enterprise-oriented, whereas poultry raised in backyards and small farms has proven to provide nutritional security worldwide. Although backyard poultry contributes more than 12% to national egg production, it is often neglected. There is a high concentration of commercial poultry egg and meat production in urban and semi-urban areas. Due to the industrial nature of their operations, the private sector is not inclined to invest in rural areas, particularly for small and landless farmers. In the commercial poultry sector, high-input and high-output birds are used to improve productivity through an integrated contract farming approach. In the case of the poorest of the poor and landless farmers, the main concerns are food security and risk spreading through subsidiary income, which is not addressed by the private sector. To solve this problem, low-input technology poultry production programs are being developed in rural areas that serve as secondary occupations providing subsistence income and improving nutritional standards, income levels, and health for rural residents.

The rural poultry program also aims to develop chickens that are more productive than native chickens, resemble native chickens, and are equally acceptable to consumers. There are four major backyard/rural poultry farming systems in India. The type of poultry farming depends on the size and management of the flock: a traditional backyard system (up to 50 birds); a semi-intensive system (50-200 birds); a small-scale intensive system (200-1000 birds); and a native chicken farming system (up to 500 birds). The choice of system depends on the market demand for the produce (eggs or meat), availability of natural food resources, and food habits of the population. Rural poultry, especially backyard poultry units, requires little hand feeding and produces handsome returns with little capital outlay. In rural areas, poultry farming not only provides income levels and employment opportunities for small farmers, such as women but also brings about necessary socioeconomic changes needed for rural prosperity and development.

The backyard/rural poultry can be classified into the following three types based on their genetic composition or type

1. Nondescript local/desi birds
2. Indigenous descript birds
3. Improved varieties

1. Nondescript local/desi birds

These non-descript local/desi birds produce fewer eggs because they have a small clutch size and have a prominent brooding instinct, but they are very adaptable to harsh climates, are disease-resistant, and are good mothers.

2. Indigenous descript birds

There are nineteen Chicken breeds in India registered with the National Bureau of Animal Genetic Resources (NBAGR). It includes Ankalsheshwar, Aseel, Busra, Chittagong, Danki, Daothigir, Ghagus, Harringhata Black, Hansli, Kadaknath, Kalasthi, Kashmir Favorolla, Kaunayen, Mewari, Miri, Nicobari, Punjab Brown and Tellicherry breeds. Kalasthi breed is vulnerable among the registered breeds. The literature also reports some lesser-known chicken breeds such as Brown Desi, Frizzle, Kumaon Hill, Naked Neck, Teni, Titri, Tripura Black, etc. These birds have small clutches and a prominent brooding instinct but are disease-resistant, resilient, and good mothers.

Advantages of native nondescript/descript Chicken

- Well adapted to traditional backyard farming
- Survive well on scavenging and leftovers with low inputs
- Disease-resistance and hardiness
- Survive in harsh conditions and protect themselves from predators
- Possess a good mothering instinct

- Compact size, coloration, alertness, and fighting abilities
- Eggs with nutritional profiles includes higher levels of various vitamins and minerals due to varied diet
- The meat is tastier when compared to commercial broilers
- Helps to preserve genetic diversity which is important for overall bio diversity
- Native chicken plays a significant role in local cultures and traditions, ceremonies, rituals and culinary practices
- Contributes to family nutrition and provides supplementary income Disadvantages of native Chicken:
- A low egg production rate
- A slower growth rate and
- Poor FCR
- Predation and theft
- Genetic diversity of native chickens is threatened by crossbreeding with commercial breeds leading to genetic erosion and loss of unique traits

3. Improved varieties

Due to the shortcomings mentioned above in native (descript/non-descript) Chickens, farmers increasingly demand hybrids suitable for rural poultry farming. To make these birds more acceptable to farmers, they must be multicolored and have brown eggs. In addition, they must be able to grow fast and produce a good number of eggs. Furthermore, they should possess predator-evasion abilities, be disease-resistant, and thrive well in village free-range conditions when fed scavengeable feed. Therefore, efforts are being focused on producing simple-housed, specific-purpose varieties with improved production profiles.

Since the mid-1990s, ICAR institutions, State Agriculture and Veterinary Universities, and other institutions have developed new varieties. The following table lists some of the varieties developed and propagated.

Sr. No.	Name of the Variety	Purpose/ Utility	Developed by
1.	CARI-SHYAMA	Egg	ICAR-CARI, Izatnagar
2.	CARI-SONALI	Egg	ICAR-CARI, Izatnagar
3.	GIRIRANI	Egg	UAS, Bengaluru
4.	GRAMALAXMI	Egg	KVASU, Pookot

Sr. No.	Name of the Variety	Purpose/ Utility	Developed by
5.	GRAMAPRIYA	Egg	ICAR-DPR, Hyderabad
6.	GRAMASREE	Egg	KVASU, Pookot
7.	KRISHNA-J	Egg	JNKVV, Jabalpur
8.	NANDANAM-1	Egg	TANUVAS, Chennai
9.	NANDANAM-2	Egg	TANUVAS, Chennai
10.	RAJASHRI	Egg	PVNRTVU, Hyderabad
11.	SATPUDA DESI	Egg	Yashwant Agri Tech., Jalgaon
12.	SWETASREE	Egg	ICAR-DPR, Hyderabad
13.	CARIBRO-DHANRAJA	Meat	ICAR-CARI, Izatnagar
14.	CARIBRO-MRITUNJAY	Meat	ICAR-CARI, Izatnagar
15.	CARIBRO-VISHAL	Meat	ICAR-CARI, Izatnagar
16.	CARIBRO-TROPICANA	Meat	ICAR-CARI, Izatnagar
17.	CARI-NIRBHEEK	Meat	ICAR-CARI, Izatnagar
18.	CARI-RAINBRO	Meat	ICAR-CARI, Izatnagar
19.	CARI-DEBENDRA	Dual	ICAR-CARI, Izatnagar
20.	GIRIRAJA	Dual	UAS, Bengaluru
21.	HITCARI	Dual	ICAR-CARI, Izatnagar
22.	JHARSIM	Dual	BAU, Ranchi
23.	KAMRUPA	Dual	AAU, Khanapara
24.	KUROILER	Dual	Kegg Farm, Delhi
25.	NARMADANIDHI	Dual	JNKVV, Jabalpur
26.	PRATAPDHAN	Dual	MPUAT, Udaipur
27.	SRINIDHI	Dual	ICAR-DPR, Hyderabad
28.	VANARAJA	Dual	ICAR-DPR, Hyderabad
29.	UPCARI	Dual	ICAR-CARI, Izatnagar

These improved varieties of chicken are readily accepted as a result of their similar appearance to local birds, low operational costs, and potential for significant profits under the existing farming systems in rural areas. These improved varieties are, therefore, the ideal substitute for native scavenging chickens in the backyard or rural poultry farming.

Interventions needed for sustainable poultry production and livelihoods in rural areas:

1. **Educating the public about the consumption of eggs and meat:** There is a need to educate children in rural schools and farming families regarding the nutritional value of eggs and meat and the importance of animal protein in the human diet. In turn, it will lead to the mass production of eggs and meat.
2. **Entrepreneurial Skill:** It is essential to provide the necessary entrepreneurial skills and knowledge to small and marginal farmers

about scientific poultry keeping to enable them to be more successful.

3. **Capacity building:** Provide training and education to farmers on poultry management practices, including nutrition, disease prevention, and biosecurity measures, to improve productivity and sustainability.
4. **Demonstrations:** Cluster-based demonstrations on the field and at the institute level are encouraged for small and marginal farmers. Method demonstrations are also necessary to provide skills in least-cost feed formulation, vaccination, deworming, medication, day-to-day management, etc.
5. **Genetic improvement:** Implement breeding programs to conserve and improve indigenous chicken breeds, focusing on traits such as disease resistance, growth rate, egg production, and adaptability to local environments.
6. **Promoting improved varieties**: Veterinarians from various State Animal Husbandry Departments, Universities, KVKs, and ICAR Institutes are required to facilitate the newly improved varieties. Veterinarians must make farmers aware of the need to rear improved varieties.
7. **Mother units for rural backyard poultry:** To overcome the problem of chick mortality, the Government has set up mother units at different locations to handle chicks up to the age of four weeks as part of the Rural Backyard Poultry Programme. However, these units need to be strengthened.
8. **Gender Empowerment**: Promote gender equality and women's empowerment in poultry production by providing women with access to training, resources, and decision-making opportunities within poultry farming enterprises.
9. **Extend input support:** As part of the input support programme, the weaker section of the society needs to give chicks, feed, medicines, feeders, drinks, and poultry rearing units or cages, as well as technical assistance for the establishment of rural poultry units. We will only provide support if they are willing to reproduce the number of chicks so they can be distributed to other weaker sections.
10. **Networking with other agencies:** It is intended to form a group among each cluster of villages and to liaise with banks, the state's animal husbandry department, wholesalers, retailers, and suppliers. Suitable farm families from villages will be identified to promote and market surplus produce in urban, peri-urban, and semi-urban areas. Farm

families will be trained in marketing. A viable relationship will also be established with societies/families who consume such products regularly. Additionally, farmers will be linked with marketers (traders and retailers) to clear surplus produce for maximum profit.

11. **Market access:** Facilitate access to markets by establishing linkages between poultry producers and buyers, supporting the development of local poultry value chains, and promoting marketing initiatives such as farmer cooperatives and collective bargaining.
12. **Encouragement for value addition and packaging:** It is also planned to train farmers on the fortification and value addition of eggs and meat and how to package and label eggs properly. Additionally, they are trained in transporting eggs and poultry meat.

The traditional rearing of 2-10 desi (nondescript/descript) birds results in lower productivity (egg and meat) and incomes. Furthermore, there is a lack of scientific knowledge about poultry rearing and disease outbreaks. Raising improved varieties to increase productivity and animal protein availability is crucial. Consequently, the activity will generate sustainable income and empower women economically and socially. By implementing the above mentioned interventions comprehensively and collaboratively, it is possible to promote sustainable poultry production and improve livelihoods for rural communities while also contributing to food security, economic development, and environmental sustainability.

21

Hygiene Management in Hatchety Unit

Vinay Singh[1]*, Asit Chakrabarti[1], Mahak Singh[2], Lopamudra Sahoo[1], Dinesh Kumar[3], K.K. Verma[4], Anil Shinde[5], Laxmi Chouhan[5], Huirem Bharati[1], Chongtham Sonia[6], Gopi M[7] and B.U. Choudhury[1]

[1]ICAR Research Complex for NEH Region, Tripura Centre Lembucherra-799210, Tripura
[2]ICAR Research Complex for NEH Region, Nagaland Centre Medziphema, Nagaland
[3]College of Veterinary Science and Animal Husbandry, BAU Kanke, Ranchi-834006
[4]Faculty of Veterinary & Animal Sciences, Institute of Agricultural Sciences Rajiv Gandhi South Campus, BHU, Barkachha, Mirzapur-231 001, U.P.
[5]College of Veterinary Science & Animal Husbandry, Jabalpur, M.P.
[6]ICAR Research Complex for NEH Region, Manipur Centre, Imphal -795004 Manipur
[7]ICAR-National Institute of Animal Nutrition and Physiology, Bengaluru Karnataka

---

Poultry hatchery is a place where the hatching egg is transformed into a one day old chick, during 21 days. The environment of a poultry hatchery is very susceptible to contamination by microorganisms which can adversely affect hatchability of the eggs and can result in embryonic deaths. E. coli, Staphylococcus species, Streptococcus species, Aspergillus fumigates and Pseudomonas species are mainly isolated from hatchery and it adversely affects chick quality and cause embryonic deaths. Poor standards of hatchery hygiene may lead ultimately to an explosion of pathogenic organisms resulting in severe economic loss. Hence hatchery hygiene is an important factor in healthy poultry production.

Sources of Contamination

1. Eggs

Even eggs look like clean in appearance it may carry thousands of bacteria and virus. One rotten egg which explodes in the setter or hatcher has the capacity to contaminate many other eggs or chicks, trays, tray carriers, trollies and fans. Contaminated eggs will lower the hatch and produce chicks with poor livability and growth.

2. Water

Water can be an important source of contamination which are used to maintain humidity in setter and hatcher by spray .

3. Air Born Infection

The air supply can introduce microorganisms to the hatchery. Improper design hatchery recycles its own waste air which is heavily contaminated with chick fluff.

4. Equipments

Improper cleaning and maintenance of equipments lead to sources of contamination in the poultry hatchery unit

5. Birds and Rodents

They are natural carriers of Salmonella and can spread in the hatchery.

6. Human beings

Employees and visitors can introduce infection to a hatchery from farms, other hatcheries, other poultry or livestock farm.

Consequences of Contamination

- Embryonic mortality
- Poor chick quality
- Low hatchability
- Poor growth rate
- High disinfectant costs
- High labour costs
- Mortality of chicks
- Economic loss

Mantainace of Hatchery Hygiene

1. Hygiene at the Layer Farm:

Hatchery hygiene begins at the layer farm. As the eggs are laid they are quickly challenged by microbes found on the floor, litter, droppings. Transfer of eggs with unsanitized hands to contaminated trays or cartons, adds to the microbial load on eggs. Rough handling of eggs added possibility to crack shells and accessing of microbes inside. Presence of rodents, birds, flies and other insects may also contaminate the eggs.

Recommendations

- Treatment of wet dropping in layer birds
- Use egg nest (mechanical or automatic) in the farm
- Frequent collection of eggs
- Remove broken and dirty egg as soon as possible
- Use clean and a dry container to collect the eggs
- Keep away biological vector such as rodents, insects, or wild birds
- Egg storage should be in a cool room (around 18°C).

Transport of Eggs

Eggs should arrive at the hatchery in the best possible condition. Control of temperature during this process is critical as changes in temperature can make the eggs sweat and increase the risk of bacteria multiplication and invasion inside the shell. Vehicle transporting the eggs should also be clean and disinfected.

2. Egg Hygiene at Hatchery Unit

On arrival in the hatchery, hatching eggs should be washed and disinfected. Proper temperature and concentration of disinfectant should maintain for egg washing . Five minutes washing is sufficient , to prevent the damage the cuticle.

Recommendations

- Use only disinfectants chemically compatible with the cleaning product.
- Washed with alkaline products (based on potassium hydroxide), to remove mainly fat and protein
- The water should be warmer than the egg contents throughout the cleaning

3. Hatchery Design

The layout and infrastructure of a hatchery have a strong influence on the efficacy of the hygiene measures. A normal hatchery contains egg storage room, fumigation room, setter room, hatcher room, chick room and store room. Hatcher room, chicks room and wash room are dirty areas of the hatchery and most of contamination spread from these areas.

Recommendations

- Strict separation of hatchery clean and dirty zones
- Proper hand washing facilities and foot dips at the entrance
- All movement should go from the clean (eggs) zone to the dirty (chicks) zone not reverse
- A positive air pressure maintain in the clean zone

4. Hatcher and Setters Hygiene

Eggs are incubated 21 days (18 days in setter and 3 days in hatcher). A specific Temperature and humidity are maintained in both to provide ideal conditions for incubation. These conditions are also optimal for growth of many pathogenic microorganisms. Better hygiene and cleaning program can prevent the growth of these microorganisms. Cleaning is most critical part of hatchery hygiene. Removal of organic debris is the best way to keep the microbial load to a minimum.

Recommendations

- Remove all the typical debris
- Cleaning should be done with a universal cleaner
- After cleaning, rinse with water and allow to dry
- Use disinfection that covers a broad spectrum with residual action
- Fumigation with formaldehyde cannot be done between 24 and 96 hours of embryonic development due to its carcinogenic nature.

5. Chick Room and Wash Room Biosecurity

- All equipment (Trays, crates and baskets) washed with alkaline detergents
- Temperatures should be higher (50-60°C), but not so high as to damage the plastic.
- Use acid, non foaming detergent to remove mineral deposits (limescale)

6. Chick Distribution

- Chicks should be placed in new boxes containing unused chick papers or chick pads.
- Vehicles and equipments used for transporting chicks for distribution should be cleaned and disinfected after each use.

7. Persons Hygiene

- Wash hands with soap and water before handling eggs and chicks.
- Use outerwear and boots in hatchery.

Monitoring of Hatchery Hygiene

Routine microbiological assessment of the hatchery is necessary to monitor the hygiene status of hatchery and it can best done by assessing air quality in different area of hatchery including setter and hatcher (air exposure plate method) and by swab sampling of surface area and culturing on trypticase soy agar (or blood agar) and MacConkey agar plates and Sabrourade Dexrose Agar. Assessing microbial load on fluff sample can also give the view of hatchery hygiene. It helps in following ways:

- Implementation of best cleaning and disinfection program
- To ensure the use of best disinfectant at in the hatchery
- To find out point of contamination in the hatchery

Conclusion

Implementation of the hygiene program in a hatchery is not only sufficient to ensure to produce a healthy chicks but also is fallow in breeding farm, broiler farm, processing unit, transport. All the person who involve in this process should be aware of all measures, facts and procedures of hygiene. A collective approach is the only way to ensure best hygienic condition in the hatchery.

References

David, D. Frame . 2010. Poultry and Game Bird Hatchery Sanitation and Biosecurity .Agriculture extension Utah State University.

Ernst, R. A., J. Glick-Smith, and A. A. Bickford.1986. Microbiological monitoring of hatchery and hatching egg sanitation. Progress in Poultry Through Research, No. 33. Cooperative Extension – University of California.

Ledoux, L. 2006. Hatchery hygiene: more than cleaning cabinet.World Poultry vol. 22 no.5.

OIE . 2010. Hygiene and disease security procedure in poultry breeding flocks and hatcheries Article 6.4.1.

22

Molting Recycling of Laying

Laxmi Chouhan, Anil Shinde, Girraj Goyal and Y.A. Rather

College of Veterinary Science and Animal Husbandry, Nanaji Deshmukh Veterinary Sciences University, Jabalpur, Madhya Pradesh, India

Introduction

Commercially laying of poultry birds carried out for a laying year or cycle after that as egg production decreases then they are usually culled when birds starts shedding of feathers. If we still keep these birds after allowing shedding and renewing of feathers birds take sufficient rest to builds up its body reserve of nutrients for next laying cycles. Their production regains 80-83% of the first laying cycle therefore recycling of laying can be carried out by shedding and renewing of feathers which is nothing but the "molting."

Naturally molting usually begins during March or April and completes by July when egg production recommences.

There are different factors that induce molting are: Physical exhaustion and fatigue, Completion of the laying cycle, Reduction of the day length, leading to reduced feeding time and resultant loss of body weight. Other some of the stress factors that may induce molting consists diseased condition, temperature extremes, nutritional imbalance, predators and poor management.

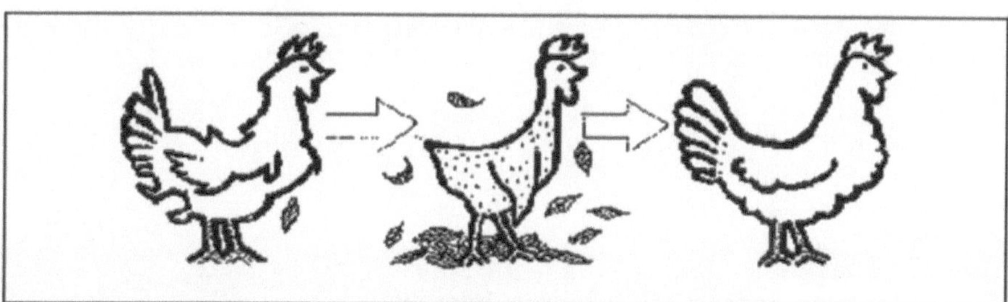

Fig.1: - Moulting process (A) (Source, Internet)

Late and early molters

"late molters" - lay for twelve to fourteen months (one laying cycle) before molt, whereas "early molters, " might begin to molt after only a couple of months in production. Early molters are usually poor producers in a flock and drop only a few feathers at a time and are slow molters as they take four to six months to complete the molt. Late molting hens are generally are the better laying hens will produce longer before molting and will shed the feathers rapidly (within two to three months). The benefit of late molters is that the loss of feathers and their replacement takes place at the same time as well as they sheds feathers as 2-3 feathers at a time. This permits the hen to return to full production sooner, thus late and rapid molter is better than early and slow molter

Order of molt

1 Head
2 Neck
3 Body (breast, back, fluff, abdomen)
4 Wing
5 Tail

In these each section of body, order of molt is regular for shedding as well as for renewing of feathers.

The molting process

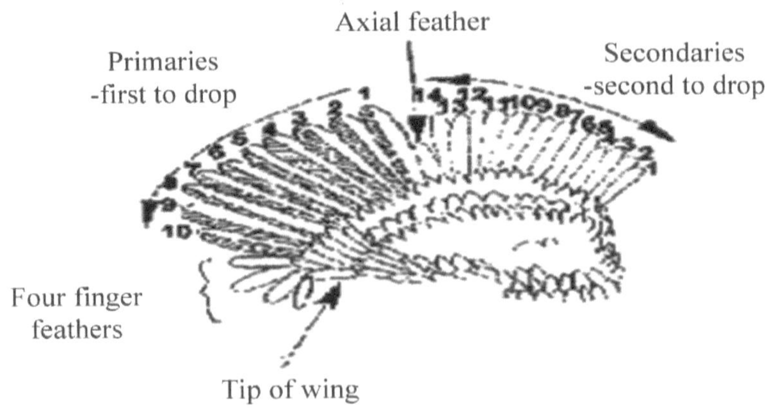

Fig.2: Moulting process (B). (Source, Internet)

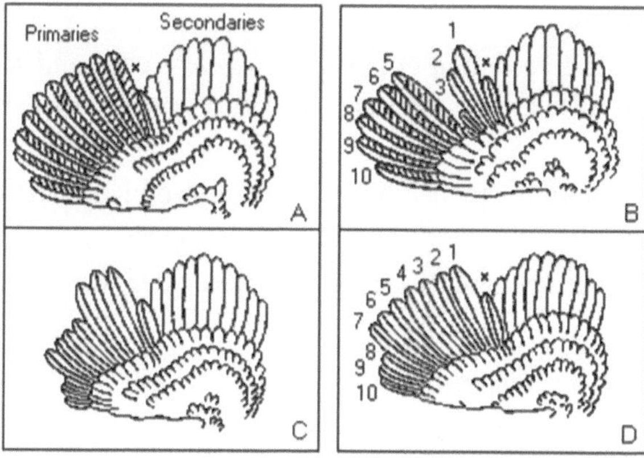

Fig. 3: Moulting process(C) (Source, Internet)

The main wing feathers consists 10 large primary which are 'flight ' feathers, a small axial feather between primary and secondary feathers and 14 secondary feathers, which are smaller and softer than the primaries. When the wing moulting starts, initially primary feathers are start to shed from the axial feather to the tip of the wing in outward direction. After that the secondaries are shed, though not in same order as the primaries. One number of primary feather drop the first then the number two and then in in sequence up to the number 10. Normally one primary feather is dropped at a time and it takes 6 weeks for new feathers to grow all new primary feathers.

Force Molting

Hens from the commercial point of view at the end of first laying year can be force molted which gives a rest period for hen to refresh body processes for the second laying cycle.

Why to Recycle /Advantages of force molting

1 When the current egg prices are low and the future egg prices are expected to be rather high it is better to molt and attain profit of next laying cycle.

2 It is cheaper to carry a bird through a molt than buy replacement pullets.

3 Fewer replacement pullets required and buying often be postponed, means saving money, time and transport.

4 Molted birds are hardier and immune as older and not much prone to disease.

Disadvantages of force molting

1 Though molted birds eat less feed than pullets, they lay less eggs and so overall, their conversion of feed into eggs and feed cost per dozen eggs is higher.

2 During the molt, they continue to eat but remain unproductive and increases cost of rearing.

3 Tenderness decreased if they are slaughtered for the table after two years of laying as age increased.

Characteristics of good molting programme

1 Entire flock should go quickly out of production.

2 Molting should ensure adequate rest.

3 It should brings back the production of flock speedily.

4 It should induce minimum however adequate stress.

5 It should be economical.

6 Mortality must be low.

7 It should be simple or easy to operate.

8 Subsequent egg production and Egg quality must be high.

Types of Recycling

1 **Two-cycle molting program**: During this one molt and two cycles of egg production carried out and the birds molted after 10-12 months of egg production.

2 **Three-cycle molting program**: Here two molt and three cycles of egg production are taken, first bird molted after 9 months of egg production and second time after 6 month of initial molt.

Force molting programme

Force molting programme administered in to the three stages

1 **Stress period** - While starting molting firstly stress imposed on birds for egg production to stop completely. Feed is withdrawn/ restricted for 12 days and restriction is also necessary for rest of this period. Careful observation necessary to limit mortality. By the end of this period body weight decreases by about 20%. Along with feed, water and light may be restricted for some hrs.

2 **Rest period** - After stress, the rest is given for 3-5 weeks. During this no egg production obtained. Rest is important to rejuvenate body processes for second cycle and throughout this only maintenance ration is given to birds.

3 **Recovery period** - Recovery of the birds starts when the hens resume laying. Peak production achieved 6-10 weeks after egg production starts. Adequate diet and 15-16 hrs light given during this period.

Comparison of first and second laying cycles

1 **Egg Production** - After molting egg production is less than first laying cycle, may be 80-83% of the first, it gives 6-8 months egg production only.

2 **Egg Quality-** Quality of egg shell and internal contents of egg improved, however after some months it decreased.

3 **Egg size-** Egg size is larger than corresponding first cycle which is one of good and major advantage of molting.

4 **Body weight-**Comparable or slightly increased than first cycle.

5 **Feed intake-** Feed intake slightly higher in second cycle.

6 **Feed potency-** Efficiency of feed is slightly poor after molt in second laying cycle compare to first cycle.

7 **Mortality-** 20% more than during the first cycle. (Normally mortality is 1% during first laying year and 1.2% during second laying year).

Same force molting programme works for males also, whereas force molting is lengthened by one or two weeks for breeders than for commercial flocks.

Programs for two cycle molting

- Conventional force molting program
- Washington force molting program
- California force molting program

Others means of causing rest to hens

Basic concept of force molting is to allow rest thus subsequent egg production increased. Besides restriction of feed, water and light, some chemical also used.

1 Methallibure- @70ppm for 13 days. Feed intake drops to 60% of normal followed by molting, egg production starts after about 8-9 weeks after the drug was first administered.

2 Enheptin- (2-amino-5-nitrothiazole) - 0.1% in diet stops egg production within 7-10 days. As long as drug fed – feed consumption suspended.

3 Others chemicals which also decrease feed consumption after feeding in diet and increase egg production after withdrawn from feed includes -

- Progesterone - 10 mg/kg feed or 15 mg inj./birds for 10 days.
- ICI compound 33828- 0.005% for 3-4 days.
- Iodine - 25-50 mg/kg feed as Potassium iodide for a week
- Zinc – 20000 ppm for 5-13 days.

23

Chicken Semen Diluents

Anil Shinde, Laxmi Chouhan, Girraj Goyal and S.H. Khan

College of Veterinary Science and Animal Husbandry, NDVSU, Jabalpur Madhya Pradesh, India

Artificial insemination (AI) technology is one of the important managemental tools for the successful poultry industry. It has several uses and a few limitations also. This technique is performed to avoid the spread of venereal diseases by natural mating and to increase the dissemination of genetic material to a large number of birds. This technique include: semen collection, semen evaluation (physical and biochemical characteristics), semen dilution and preservation and deposition of semen in the female genitalia. Semen dilution is one of the most critical components of AI technology. Several suitable semen dilutors are reviewed for low temperature storage up to around 48 hours. The chicken semen dilutors available so far have complex composition and require many ingredients. They are also difficult to prepare at farm level. These dilutors can keep the spermatozoa viable at lower temperatures for reasonably long periods by suppressing the activities of sperm temporarily. It is known that undiluted raw fowl semen stored in vitro usually decreases sperm motility and the fertilizing capacity within 1h after collection. Therefore, to store cockerel semen, the type of diluent and storage temperature is very crucial.

Semen Diluents

Diluents are buffered salt solutions used to extend semen, maintain the viability of spermatozoa in vitro, and maximize the number of hens that can be inseminated. Semen dilution or extension is important since poultry semen is viscous and highly concentrated, containing 6 (roosters) to 12 (toms) billion spermatozoa/ml. Semen diluents are based on the biochemical composition of chicken semen. Glutamic acid, the most prominent anionic constituent of avian seminal plasma, became a standard component of diluents. There are many extender /diluents available for chicken semen, both with published recipes and commercially available products. Several investigators have compared the composition of various diluents and summarized fertility data across. What is evident from these reviews is that there is no standard diluent for poultry semen and that studies are so variable in experimental design including time of insemination, vaginal depth and frequency of AI, number of spermatozoa inseminated and duration of fertility analyzed that discerning the benefits of different diluents is difficult.

There are basic characteristics common to nearly all diluents: factors to maintain pH, osmolarity and provide an energy source for spermatozoa. The pH of a diluent can affect the metabolic rate and motility of spermatozoa. Buffering agents, consisting of a mixture of an acid and its conjugate base are formulated into a diluent to limit changes in pH. These usually include the mixture of phosphates, citrates and/or organic zwitter ionic molecules such as *N*, *N*-bis (2-hydroxyethyl)-2-aminoethane sulfonic acid (BES) and *N*-Tris (hydroxymethyl) methyl-2-aminoethane sulfonic acid (TES) in poultry diluents. Zwitter ionic molecules are important in diluents for chicken semen because of lactic acid build up with increased storage time which can lower the diluent pH. Chicken and turkey spermatozoa can tolerate a pH range of 6.0–8.0. Diluent pH alteres the motility and metabolic rate of spermatozoa. For example, a low pH reduces motility, lactic acid production, oxygen uptake in chicken spermatozoa, whereas high pH increases metabolic rates in vitro. For 24h storage of chicken semen, pH of 6.8 and 7.1 improved survival over diluents with pH of 5.8 and 7.4.

Poultry spermatozoa can maintain fertilizing ability in diluents with osmolarities ranging from 250 to 460 mosm/kg H_20. When spermatozoa are placed in a solution of low osmolarity, the net movement of water into the sperm cells causes them to swell. In a hyperosmotic solution, spermatozoa loose water and shrink down. This physical property is the basis of commonly used spermatozoa stress tests discussed in subsequent sections. In hypoosmotic conditions spermatozoa display increased incidence of bent necks, a defect frequently found in diluted chicken semen, which is negatively correlated with fertility. For the development of diluents and storage systems for poultry semen important is the physiological differences and metabolic requirements of spermatozoa from different species. Chicken spermatozoa are metabolically competent in aerobic and anaerobic environments in vitro. In contrast, turkey spermatozoa require high levels of oxygen to survive. Aerobic metabolism requires the aeration of semen which is generally accomplished by placing diluted semen in a flask to maximize surface to volume ratio and placing the flask on a rotary shaker. More recently, other methods to maximize and control oxygen supply to semen have been investigated. These include the addition of perfluoro chemicals, compounds that chelate oxygen and the development of environmentally controlled capsules that regulate temperature and oxygen concentration.

The diluents or extenders used in poultry production must have buffers to prevent changes or stabilize the semen pH. The commonly used buffers are Tris, sodium citrate and sodium phosphate. The sperm membrane is, as already mentioned, also susceptible to changes in temperature, and this may affect the movement of the sperm, causing deterioration in semen quality. Care must therefore be taken to maintain the diluted semen at the prescribed temperatures. The diluents must be isotonic as osmotic pressure created in the solution could be detrimental to the sperm e.g. dehydration of the cell. Diluents or extenders must also protect the sperm against cold shock injury during freezing, provide the necessary nutrients for sperm metabolism, and contain penicillin and streptomycin to control microbial contaminants. Further diluents must contain a cryoprotectant to protect the sperm from injury during freezing and thawing, and must preserve the viability of the sperm, with a minimum drop in overall fertility.

Importance of dilution

- To inseminate a greater number of females than with a quantity of undiluted semen.
- To transport semen from one place to another place without reduction in its fertilizing ability.
- To store semen beyond a hour.
- To utilize small volume of semen of semen containing sufficient spermatozoa from a valuable proven sire for insemination.
- To reduce the cost of AI by maintenance of a smaller number of males.
- To solve the problem of germplasm preservation by extending from some valuable sires and storing it for extended periods of time.

Short Term Cockerel Semen Preservation

Semen diluents are currently being used for both short- and long-term storage of domestic fowl semen. These extenders are being commercialized to improve the general reproductive effectiveness of the cockerels and lower the cost of AI. The semen diluents development initially began with the use of NaCl (Normal saline) solutions. Now complex diluents containing different osmotic regulators, energy sources and buffers are being used. Short term (hours to days at a temperature of -4°C) fowl semen storage requires the suspension of sperm in a suitable extender to maintain the sperm viability, in vitro.

Table 1: Different dilutors: some of the commonly used diluents are as follows

Ingredients	BPSE	Lakes	Egg Yolk
Fructose	5.00	10.00	-
$MgCl_2$	0.34	0.68	-
Trisodium citrate	0.64	1.28	-
Sodium acetate	4.30	8.51	-
Sodium glutamate	8.67	19.20	-
Glucose	-	-	42.50
Egg yolk ml	-	-	150
NaCl	-	-	-
TES	1.95	-	-
Potassium Mono phosphate	0.75	-	-
Dipotassium hydrogen phosphate	12.70	-	-
Whole milk	-	-	-
PH	7.5	7.0	6.9
Osmotic Pressure (mos/kgH_2O)	333	375	327

Modified Ringer's Solution: - with the following composition

- Sodium chloride (68g),
- Potassium chloride (17.33g),
- Calcium chloride (6.42g),
- Magnesium sulphate (2.50g),
- Sodium bicarbonate (24.50g) and
- Distilled water, can be used to dilute poultry semen (Martin, 2004).

Beltsville Poultry Semen Extender (BPSE)

BPSE was developed by Sexton (1977), (Table 2) being one of the first people to discover the importance of the dilution of the insemination dose required for optimum fertility following short term semen storage in poultry.

Table 2: The composition of the Beltsville Poultry Semen Extender (Sexton, 1977)

Component	Level g/l	Primary function
Dipotassium phosphate	12.70	Buffer
Sodium glutamate	8.61	Chelator
Fructose	5.00	Metabolic substrate
Sodium acetate	4.30	Osmotic balance
TES*	1.95	Buffer
Potassium citrate	0.64	Osmotic balance
Monopotassium phosphate	0.65	Buffer
Magnesium chloride	0.34	Osmotic balance

*N-Tris (Hydroxymethyl) Methyl-2-Aminoethane sulfonic acid

Table 3: Semen Extender & their particulars

Semen Extender	Dilution Rate	Max. holding time (hrs)	Holding temp. (°C)	Insemination dose
Modified Ringers Solution	3	4	10	0.1 ml
Lakes Solution	2	8	10	0.1 ml
EYCB	5	24-48	5	0.3 ml (duck)
Modified Tyrode's Solution	3	0.25	37	0.05 ml
BPSE	4	-	5	20 milli.

Table 4: CARI Diluents: CARI, Izatnagar also have developed some of the semen diluents with following characteristics

	Simple Diluents	Complex Diluents
Composition	**Phosphate Buffer, Sugar, Sodium glutamate**	**Phosphate Buffer, Sugar, Sodium Glutamate, Sod. Acetate Tris, Tri Potta. Citrate**
PH:	7.2	7.2
Osmotic Press.	390	338
Dilution Rate	1:3	1:3
Holding Temp.	2-5 °C	2-5 °C
Store Temp.	24 hrs	24 hrs

Conclusion

- Semen diluent facilitates the even distribution of spermatozoa to obtain optimal fertility.
- It helps to lower the cost of production by reducing number of males needed for AI.
- It also permits the transportation and distribution of desirable genes

throughout the world.

- Currently semen dilution has most of its commercial application in the breeding of turkeys where the practice of AI is obligatory.
- Semen dilutor will have little further application until the technique of AI is more.
- Semen diluents should be developed for alternate poultry species.
- Technique of cryo-preservation of avian semen should be strengthen.

24

Organic Poultry Farming Navigating Opportunities, Challenges, and Certification in India

Monika. M[1]., Rokade. J.J[2]., Sonale, N.S[2]., Prasad Wadajkar[2] and S. KerKetta[1]

[1]ICAR-Indian Agricultural Research Institute, Hazaribagh, Jharkhand-825405
[2]ICAR-Central Avian Research Institute, Bareilly, Uttar Pradesh -243122

Organic farming has undergone rapid growth in recent years across various agricultural and livestock sectors, including poultry production. The escalation of health concerns stemming from the presence of numerous medications and pesticide residues in conventional products has underscored the importance of ensuring the quality of egg and meat products. In this global context, there is a notable surge in demand for organic meat, prompting nations to explore organic poultry production. The term "organic" pertains to the method by which livestock and agricultural products are cultivated and processed, prioritizing the avoidance of agrochemicals such as synthetic pesticides and fertilizers. While the absence of chemical inputs serves as a fundamental aspect of non-chemical farming, organic production encompasses a broader spectrum of considerations. It emphasizes animal health and welfare, promotes environmentally sound practices, and prioritizes product quality. In contrast, conventional production primarily centres on cost reduction and maximizing output by focusing on factors such as weight gain and feed efficiency (Sundrum, 2006).

Organic livestock farming is particularly well-suited to Indian conditions due to the indigenous technical knowledge and practices followed by Indian farmers. However, despite the substantial poultry population in India, the transition from conventional to organic poultry farming has been relatively slow. Nonetheless, a modest shift in this direction has the potential to create a substantial market for both domestic consumption and export. Within the realm of organic farming, adherence to defined standards in production and handling is paramount. The primary objectives of organic poultry production encompass sustainable resource utilization, environmental protection, and meticulous animal care. According to the Food and Agriculture Organization (FAO), organic farming is defined as a distinct production management system designed to promote and enhance the health of the agroecosystem. This includes considerations for biodiversity, biological cycles, and soil biological activity. Achieving these goals involves the utilization of on-farm agronomic, biological, and mechanical methods, replacing synthetic off-farm inputs. Organic farming is characterized as an integrated agricultural approach with the overarching goal of establishing humane, environmentally sustainable, and economically viable agricultural production systems. A key objective of organic farming is to generate crops that meet acceptable standards for both livestock and human nutrition while safeguarding them from pests and diseases, thereby ensuring optimal returns on human and other resources invested. (Jagmeet and anand. 2023) Emphasizing holistic health management and fostering a biologically active soil, organic poultry farming aims to enhance bird health and contribute to environmental sustainability. By employing this agricultural technique, all pesticides, hormones, antibiotics, and other contaminants are entirely eliminated from the final product. These attributes have led to a significant demand for organic products, particularly among the educated and health-conscious consumer population.

The growing awareness of health and well-being among individuals has led to a shift in preferences from conventionally produced food to organically grown alternatives. Worldwide, organic livestock farming is gaining rapid popularity, driven by the escalating demand for organic milk, meat, and egg products, coupled with increased consumer awareness regarding the quality of these products. The prevalence of various pesticides, insecticides, chemicals, drugs, and hormone residues has been linked to lifestyle-related issues such as diabetes and cancer. The higher incidence of cancer in developed countries, attributed to intensive and mechanized agriculture, underscores the urgency for organic alternatives. Other driving reasons may include increasing intake of bread products and high protein diets advocated by gym trainers. However, the high expense of organic feed may pose additional impediments to market expansion. Furthermore, a lack of technological advances and a limited supply of organic feed ingredients will act as significant barriers, reducing the organic poultry feed market's growth rate. With this background, the present chapter gives in detail knowledge about organic farming in poultry, its scope and challenges in India and finally the certification procedures.

Status of Organic Poultry Farming

The organic poultry market has experienced robust growth in recent years, with its size increasing steadily, and this growth is projected to continue into the future. In 2023, the organic poultry market was valued at $8.44 billion, and by 2024, it is expected to reach $8.86 billion, reflecting a compound annual growth rate (CAGR) of 5.0%. This growth in the historic period can be attributed to several factors including low interest rates, rising spendable incomes, increased demand for quality and sustainability, the adoption of slow-growing chicken breeds, and a growing awareness of environmental concerns, as well as the expansion of emerging markets. Looking ahead, the organic poultry market is forecasted to maintain its upward trend, reaching $10.54 billion by 2028, with a CAGR of 4.4%. This growth in the forecast period is anticipated due to technological advancements, stricter political regulations, and heightened awareness of the health benefits associated with organic poultry consumption. Notable trends expected to shape the market in the forecast period include the development and investment in new ready-to-eat variants of organic poultry products to expand product portfolios and meet increasing demand, as well as to remain competitive.

Organic Poultry production: The global scenario

- 69.8 million ha land in 181 countries, over 2.9 Million producers grow organic foods. USD 97.00 billion global market for organic products. Over 87 countries now have an organic legislation.
- Organic milk production currently stands at 4.4million metric tons (European Union: 4.1 million), constituting more than 2.8 percent of the European Union 's milk production from dairy cows in 2016
- As per USDA, sales of organic broilers in US in 2017 rose by 78% to $750m, making it the largest growing market in the organic sector, while organic egg sales rose by 11% to $816m

India: An organic Success Story

- With 8,35,200 producers India continues to be No. 1 country followed by Uganda (210,352) and Mexico (210,000)
- India ranks 9th in area under Organic agriculture in the world
- Area under organic certification process 3.56 million Hectare (2017-18). India produced around 1.70 million MT (2017-18) of certified organic products. The total volume of export during 2017-18 was 4.58 lakh MT. India exported organic products worth Rs 5151 Crore (over US $ 757 million) in 2018-19, from Rs 3453 Crore in 2017-18 (US$

515 million) registering an increase of about 49 %. In terms of export value realization Oilseeds (47.6%) lead among the products followed by Cereals and millets (10.4%), Plantation crop products such as Tea and Coffee (8.96%), Dry fruits (8.88%), Spices and condiments (7.76%) and others.

- There are 28 Accredited Certification Bodies under NPOP
- Increasing support of government agencies apart from NGOs and Private sector
- Sikkim has converted its entire cultivable land (more than 76000 ha) under organic certification.
- Indian organic products are welcome in EU & US and other countries around the world-global recognition! India exported organic products worth Rs 5151 Crore (over US $ 757 million) in 2018-19, from Rs 3453 Crore in 2017-18 (US$ 515 million) registering an increase of about 49 %. In XII plan, the GOI has launched Paramparagat Krishi Vikas Youjana, under which Rs. 300 Crores (Union Budget 2015-16) were allocated to promote organic agriculture including organic animal husbandry. The organic livestock and poultry standards have also been notified for implementation since 1st June, 2015 (APEDA, 2015).

However, there is substantial potential for the country to transition from conventional to organic poultry production. Such a shift could not only cater to the domestic market but also create opportunities for exports. Given India's abundant resources, the organic poultry sector holds considerable promise for expansion, both domestically and in the export market.

Concept of Organic Poultry Production

Organic poultry farming follows a unique production management system as defined by the FAO/WHO Codex Alimentarius Commission. It aims to promote and enhance the health of agro ecosystems, including biodiversity, biological cycles, and soil biological activity. This is achieved through the use of on-farm agronomic, biological, and mechanical methods, excluding all synthetic off-farm inputs. The primary goal of organic farming is to establish and maintain interdependence between soil, plants, animals, and their environment, creating a sustainable agro-ecological system using local resources. Unlike conventional farming, organic poultry farming minimizes reliance on external inputs such as fertilizers and antibiotics, instead emphasizing ecosystem management. Livestock, including poultry, play a vital role in this system by contributing to the agricultural cycle. Transitioning from conventional to organic management requires a careful and gradual approach, involving a specific period known as the "conversion period." This period marks the time between the start of organic management on the farm and the certification of the livestock farm and its products. In organic poultry farming, preference is given to local breeds, and great care is taken to provide an environment that allows birds to exhibit their natural behaviours. This approach aligns with the principles of organic farming, emphasizing sustainability, biodiversity, and the well-being of both animals and the environment.

Foundational Aspects of Organic Poultry Farming

Breeding: Organic farming necessitates the selection of local and indigenous breeds, as genetically engineered breeds are not deemed organic. Natural reproductive techniques must be employed. Birds should be sourced from production units adhering to organic standards or from farms where parents are raised organically. While vaccination against common diseases is permitted, genetically modified vaccines are prohibited. Introducing non-organic poultry is only permissible under specific conditions, such as operating an organic poultry farm for the first time, introducing a special breed, or renewing the farm's herd.

Housing: The primary objective of organic housing and management standards is to allow poultry birds to express their natural behaviors with minimal stress. Birds should have access to the outdoors, exercise areas, shade, and direct sunlight suitable to their life stage, climate, and environment. Clean, dry bedding and shelter conducive to natural behaviors, comfort, and exercise opportunities should be provided. Protecting birds from predators is a key concern, as caging is not permitted in organic poultry production. Birds should be raised under a deep litter system. Artificial lighting can be used within the parameters set by certification agencies. Typically, birds are raised for a period of around 81 days in the organic meat sector.

Conversion Period

The initiation of organic poultry farming involves a distinct phase known as the "conversion period." This period marks the duration between the onset of organic management on the farm and the attainment of certification for both the farm and its products. The conversion period commences with the initial inspection. It is imperative that both the land and poultry undergo conversion simultaneously. However, if the conversion of land and poultry is not simultaneous, then the poultry must undergo a specific period of rearing, with a minimum duration of raising meat poultry starting from the second day of hatching and six weeks for eggs, as stipulated by the organic board, before the products can be marketed as organic.

Feeding

Organic poultry farming mandates the provision of high-quality organically grown feed to the birds. No more than 20% of the feed should originate from non-organic sources. With the exception of vitamin and mineral supplements, all ingredients must possess organic certification. The diet should be presented in a manner that enables birds to express natural feeding behaviors and meet their digestive requirements. Poultry should be provided with organically produced concentrated balanced feed rations. Utilization of homegrown protein sources like peas, beans, and rapeseed is encouraged, with specific inclusion rates for meat birds and laying hens. Sprouted pulses serve as an excellent source of vitamins and can be used to replace synthetic amino acids. Preferably, trace minerals incorporated into the diets should be organic. Essential amino acid requirements can be met through the inclusion of organic soybean, skim milk powder, potato protein, maize gluten, among others. Overfeeding must be avoided. Continuous access to ample supplies of drinking water of standard quality, free from residues, is essential. Regular water testing should be conducted and recorded. The feed used must not contain animal products, growth-promoting hormones, urea, or manure. Additionally, it should not include any additives or supplements that violate regulations set by the Food and Drug Administration, including those containing antibiotics or ionophores.

Healthcare

In the realm of organic farming, the foundation of healthcare and management is cantered around practices that prioritize the well-being of poultry, thereby enhancing their natural resistance to diseases and infections. Maintaining clean grazing areas and dry litter plays a pivotal role in preventing a multitude of health-related issues. While the use of antibiotics is discouraged, vaccinations are permissible when the anticipation of diseases arises. Embracing natural remedies such as homeopathy and ayurveda is encouraged in organic poultry production.

Organic poultry producers are tasked with implementing preventative healthcare measures, which include

- Selecting poultry species and types resilient to prevalent diseases and parasites, tailored to specific site conditions.
- Providing a nutritionally balanced feed ration, encompassing essential vitamins, minerals, proteins, amino acids, fatty acids, and energy sources.

- Establishing appropriate housing, pasture conditions, and sanitation practices to mitigate the occurrence and spread of diseases and parasites.
- Ensuring conditions conducive to exercise, freedom of movement, and stress reduction, aligning with the natural behavior of the species (for instance, avoiding caged environments for laying hens).
- Conducting physical alterations, when necessary, to promote poultry welfare, with measures taken to minimize pain and stress.
- Administering vaccines and veterinary biologics as part of the overall healthcare regimen.

Record Keeping

Effective record keeping is paramount in organic poultry farming, serving as a cornerstone for management practices. It involves systematic documentation of activities, observations, and inferences for future reference. Records encompass a wide range of aspects, including breeding data, registers detailing the sources of animal procurement, organic feed ingredients, feed supplements, and additives, as well as formulation records for organic feed. Additionally, records include documentation of poultry pasture management, inventory of healthcare and sanitation products, monthly flock records for organic egg layers and meat poultry, summaries of poultry slaughter and sales, and records of egg packing and sales on a monthly basis.

Persuasive Arguments for Opting for Organic Poultry

Healthier Choices: Organic poultry products are free from antibiotics, added hormones, and GMO feed, ensuring that consumers receive a healthier option without unwanted additives.

Environmental Benefits: Organic poultry farming practices prioritize sustainability and environmental stewardship, minimizing the use of synthetic chemicals and promoting biodiversity.

Animal Welfare: Organic poultry farming emphasizes humane treatment, allowing birds to roam freely outdoors and express natural behaviors, leading to improved welfare standards.

Reduced Chemical Exposure: By avoiding synthetic pesticides and fertilizers, organic poultry production reduces the risk of chemical residues in food products, benefiting both consumers and the environment.

Support for Sustainable Agriculture: Choosing organic poultry supports farmers who utilize sustainable farming practices, promoting soil health, water conservation, and long-term agricultural sustainability.

Higher Nutritional Value: Organic poultry products have been shown to contain higher levels of certain nutrients, including omega-3 fatty acids and antioxidants, due to the birds' natural diet and healthier living conditions.

Safer Food Supply: Organic poultry production adheres to strict standards and regulations, ensuring a safer and more transparent food supply chain for consumers.

Protection of Natural Resources: Organic farming methods prioritize the conservation of natural resources such as soil, water, and air, helping to mitigate environmental degradation and climate change.

Ethical Considerations: By choosing organic poultry, consumers support ethical farming practices that prioritize animal welfare, sustainability, and social responsibility.

Personal Health Benefits: Consuming organic poultry products can contribute to better overall health and well-being, as they are free from potentially harmful chemicals and antibiotics commonly found in conventional poultry production

Breed/ variety developed for rural poultry farming which can use for organic poultry farming

Sr.	Breed/ variety	Type	Institution	Remarks
1.	Vanaraja	Dual	PDR, Hyderabad	Better immune competence
2.	Giriraja	Dual	PDR, Hyderabad	Suitable for meat& egg
3.	CARI Nirbhik	Dual	CARI, Izzatnagar	Suitable for meat& egg
4.	CARI Shayama	Dual	CARI, Izzatnagar	Suitable for meat& egg
5.	CARI Hitcari	Dual	CARI, Izzatnagar	Suitable for meat& egg
6.	Nico- rock	Dual	CARI, Portblair	Suitable for hot humid costal area
7.	Krishna Priya	Dual	KAU, Manuthy	Suitable for meat& egg
8.	Gram Priya	Egg	PDR, Hyderabad	Suitable for egg
9.	Nishibari	Egg	CARI, Portblair	Suitable for hot humid areas
10.	Rajashree	Egg	SVVU, Hyderabad	Suitable for egg
11.	Pratapadhan	Dual	MPUAT, Udaipur	Reasonable with local birds of Rajasthan
12.	Kamarupa	Dual	AAU, Guwahati	High survival rate
13.	Srinidhi	Dual	PDR, Hyderabad	High egg producer under farm as well as backyard condition

Challenges in Organic Poultry Farming

Challenges includes

1. **High Initial Investment:** Transitioning from conventional to organic poultry farming often requires a significant initial investment. Organic farming practices, such as providing larger outdoor spaces and organic feed, can be costlier than conventional methods.

2. **Lack of Awareness and Education:** Many farmers in India may not be fully aware of the principles and requirements of organic poultry farming. Education and training are essential to ensure that farmers understand the necessary practices and standards.
3. **Certification Process:** Obtaining organic certification can be a complex and expensive process. Farmers need to comply with strict organic standards and undergo inspections, which can be a barrier, especially for small-scale producers.
4. **Limited Availability of Organic Feed:** Finding a consistent and affordable supply of organic feed can be a challenge. Most conventional poultry farms rely on conventional feed, and organic feed options may be limited and costly.
5. **Disease Management:** Organic poultry farms often rely on preventive measures rather than antibiotics for disease management. This can be challenging in India, where disease outbreaks are common due to factors like overcrowding and poor sanitation.
6. **Market Access:** While the demand for organic poultry products is increasing, accessing organic markets can be difficult. Farmers may face challenges in marketing their products and finding buyers willing to pay premium prices.
7. **Land Availability**: Providing adequate outdoor space for birds to roam and forage is a requirement of organic poultry farming. In densely populated areas of India, finding suitable and for this purpose can be challenging.
8. **Climate Variability:** India's diverse climate can pose challenges for organic poultry farming. Extreme temperatures and monsoon rains can affect bird health and require additional management practices.
9. **Competition with Conventional Poultry:** Conventional poultry farming in India is dominant and often more profitable due to higher production volumes and lower costs. This competition can make it difficult for organic poultry to thrive.
10. **Transportation and Infrastructure:** Maintaining the integrity of organic products during transportation and storage can be challenging in regions with limited infrastructure.

Despite these challenges, the interest in organic poultry farming in India is growing due to increasing consumer demand for organic and ethically produced food products. Overcoming these obstacles may require government support, increased awareness, and investment in organic agriculture infrastructure and research to make organic poultry farming a more viable and sustainable option for Indian farmers.

Certification for Organic Poultry Farming

Certification for organic poultry farming in India is a rigorous process that involves meeting specific standards and requirements set by accredited certification bodies. Here are the steps to apply for certification of organic poultry farming in India:

1. ***Understand Organic Standards:*** Familiarize yourself with the organic standards and regulations applicable in India. In India, the National Program for Organic Production (NPOP) sets the guidelines for organic certification. These standards cover various aspects of organic farming, including poultry farming.
2. ***Prepare Your Farm:*** Ensure that your poultry farm complies with organic farming practices and meets the NPOP standards. This includes providing outdoor access for birds, using organic feed, avoiding synthetic chemicals, and following humane treatment practices.
3. ***Select a Certification Body:*** Choose a reputable certification body accredited by the Agricultural and Processed Food Products Export Development Authority (APEDA) or other relevant authorities. Some well-known organic certification bodies in India include Organic Farmers and Growers (India) Pvt. Ltd., Ecocert India, and OneCert International Pvt. Ltd.
4. ***Contact the Certification Body:*** Reach out to the chosen certification body and request an application form and information about the certification process. You may need to pay an application fee.
5. *Complete the Application Form:* Fill out the application form provided by the certification body. This form will typically ask for information about your farm, practices, and the type of organic poultry you intend to raise.
6. ***Document Compliance:*** Gather all necessary documents and records, including farm layout plans, records of feed sources, documentation of practices, and any other information required by the certification body. Ensure that you have maintained these records for the required duration.
7. ***On-Site Inspection*:** The certification body will conduct an on-site inspection of your poultry farm. During this visit, inspectors will assess your compliance with organic standards, including the living conditions of birds, feed sources, pest control methods, and record-keeping practices.

8. ***Corrective Actions*:** If any non-compliance issues are identified during the inspection, you will need to take corrective actions to address them and bring your farm into compliance with organic standards.
9. ***Certification Decision*:** After the inspection and review of your application and records, the certification body will make a decision regarding your organic certification. If your farm meets all the requirements, you will be granted organic certification.
10. ***Annual Inspections:*** Organic certification is not a one-time process. You will need to undergo annual inspections to maintain your organic certification. These inspections ensure that you continue to meet organic standards.
11. ***Pay Certification Fees:*** Be prepared to pay certification fees to the certification body, which cover the cost of inspections, reviews, and administrative expenses.
12. ***Market Your Organic Products:*** Once certified, you can market your organic poultry and poultry products as "organic." Make sure to follow labelling and marketing guidelines set by the certification body.

Remember that the process of organic certification can be complex and time-consuming. It's essential to maintain detailed records, maintain compliance with organic standards, and work closely with the chosen certification body to ensure a smooth certification process. Certification is a valuable asset for marketing organic poultry products and meeting the growing demand for organic and sustainable food in India and beyond.

Conclusion

Organic poultry farming represents a sustainable and ethical approach to poultry production that prioritizes animal welfare, environmental conservation, and consumer health. The global demand for organic poultry products is on the rise, driven by increasing awareness of the health and environmental benefits associated with organic farming practices. India, with its rich agricultural heritage and vast resources, has the potential to become a leader in organic poultry production. Despite facing challenges such as high initial investment, lack of awareness, and limited availability of organic feed, the organic poultry sector in India is experiencing significant growth. Government support, increased awareness, and investment in infrastructure and research are essential for overcoming these challenges and fostering the expansion of organic poultry farming in the country. Certification for organic poultry farming is a rigorous process that ensures compliance with organic standards and regulations. By obtaining organic certification, farmers can access lucrative markets and meet the growing demand for organic and ethically produced food products. In Nutshell organic poultry farming offers a promising pathway towards sustainable agriculture, healthier food choices, and economic prosperity for Indian farmers. With the right support and commitment, organic poultry production can thrive, benefiting both farmers and consumers alike.

25

Avian Sex Reversal Current Status and Future Prospects

Kurva Shiva Kumar, Sagar Raghunath Khandagale, Jagbir Singh Tyagi, Matin Ansari, Sirjauddin and Gautham Kolluri

Division of Avian Physiology and Reproduction, ICAR-Central Avian Research Institute, Izatnagar-243122, Bareilly, Uttar Pradesh

Poultry is one of the most emerging growth components of Indian agriculture, with egg and meat production rising at the rate of 8-10% per year when compared to crop production (1.5 - 2% each year). In India, the poultry population stood at 851.81 million in the 20th livestock census, an increase of 16.8% over the 19th census. Poultry sectors contribute 1% of national GDP and 25% in livestock GDP (FAO, 2021). According to DAHD's 2022 report, our nation produces 122.05 billion eggs and 4.47 million tonnes of poultry meat altogether. India ranks eighth in terms of total meat production and third in terms of total egg production (DAHD, 2022). In India, the production of poultry meat makes up more than half of the total meat production (Singh, 2020). Backyard poultry increased by over 45.78% with 317.07 million in 2019, while commercial poultry increased by over 4.5% by 534.74 million in 2019 (20th Livestock Census). Poultry meat production increased by 6.86%, however egg production increased by 6.19% (BAHS, 2022). With the growing population and the ever-increasing proportion of meat consumers, the need for more production is there. The current per capita availability of eggs is 90 eggs and 3.8 kg of poultry meat (DADH, 2021), compared to the ICMR recommended consumption of 180 eggs and 10.8 kg of meat per person per year.

In layer industry, male birds are typically eliminated, meaning that only female birds are needed, which poses serious issues for both the economy and animal welfare (Doran *et al.*, 2017). For the poultry industry, the ability to produce monosexual lines of birds—that is, exclusively females—would be extremely valuable. Over 180 million male chicks are killed each year in India, while over 7.0 billion newborn male chicks are slaughtered globally each year (Galli *et al.*, 2016; Alin *et al.*, 2019). Farmers are particularly interested in male broiler chicks because they grow quicker than female chicks and have a higher feed conversion rate (Schmid *et al.*, 2015).

Avian Sex Reversal

The term "sex reversal" is typically used to characterise individuals who have extra-gonadal and gonadal sexual phenotypes that are the reverse of their sex chromosome (A T. Major, 2016). Most often, zoo and domesticated birds experience sex reversal. Bird genera include *Gallus gallus, Aas boschas, Perdix cinerea, Pavo spp, Phasianus spp, Columbo livia, Meleagris spp., Anas penelope, Aythya marila, Melanitta nigra, Mergus serrator, and Tetrao urogallus* (Forbes, 1947). The condition of atypical sexual development in poultry was first described by Aristotle (Taber, 1964).

The reversal of sex in animals can be attributed to various factors such as temperature, salinity, water pH, and social interaction (Baroiller, 2001). However, in birds, sex reversal is caused by the asymmetry or unique laterality of the gonad during the development of the male and female genitalia, where a higher number of primordial gametes migrate to the left gonad than to the right (Smith and Sinclair, 2004). In domestic chickens (Gallus domesticus), sex reversal is well-known and has been documented in both natural and experimental (Thomas and Marion, 2003). In birds, alterations in the synthesis or activity of oestrogen can cause a very strong reversal of sex (Vaillant *et al.*, 200; Ayers *et al.*, 2013c).

History of Sex Identification & Avian reproductive system

According to Anaxagoras 'theory of sex determination' the sex of the progeny is decided by the father; females develop from the left testicle's sperm and males from the right. In his article "On the Origin of Animals," he observed that males had the superior element of fire, while females have an excess of the cold element of water. Empedocles (490–430 BC) proposed four elements "fire, water, air, and earth" in men are hotter than women (Lesky, 1951). William Harvey postulated that all species, including humans and viviparous animals, descended from an egg in his 1651 "Aphorism ex ovo omnia" (from the egg everything). Nettie Stevens and Edmund Wilson argued that sex is determined by chromosomes.

The genus Galloanserae includes chickens (amniotes) (Clarie Hirst, 2017). They have 39 diploid (2n) chromosomes, which are made up of 29 pairs of microchromosomes and 10 pairs of macrochromosomes (which vary in size, shape, and binding pattern) of chromosomes Z and W. Bird sex identification is more challenging when the birds are nestlings, but it is crucial for behavioural ecology, genetics, evolutionary biology, and conservation biology—particularly when it comes to captive breeding endangered species (Ito *et al.,* 2003). While female birds (ZW) are heterogametic, with the left gonad developing into an ovary and the right gonad remaining vestigial, male birds (ZZ) have two identical sex chromosomes with a pair of testes (Jeong, 2009; Lambeth, 2012). Sex reversal is caused by direct hormonal and genetic pathways, however in mammals, only the genetic component (Smith, 2016).

Avian Sex Differentiation

In birds, sexual differentiation is a crucial aspect of sexual development that is mediated by direct hormonal and genetic pathways. In certain situations, sexual differentiation-regulating genes can also become active in other organs, such the brain, even prior to gonadal sexual differentiation. The undifferentiated or so-called bipotent gonad, and the genital ridge (Zhang *et al.,* 2010; Ayers *et al.,* 2013b). According to Hamburger and Hamilton's technique, a chicken embryo grows over a period of 21 days and experiences 45 distinct phases (HH, 1951). The embryonic gonads develop on the ventromedial surface of the developing embryonic kidneys (mesonephros). The gonads start to develop at E3.5, and the intermediate mesoderm matures into the urogenital tissues (Kuroiwa, 2017). The gonads are thought to be "bipotential" up until approximately E6.5, implying that they are predisposed to differentiate into either the testes or the ovaries. Most of the undifferentiated gonads, also called genital ridges, are composed of the outer cortex and inner medulla in both sexes (Smith, 2011; Nandi, 2014). Gonadal precursors emerge from coelomic epithelium and mesonephros precursors at about E2 (Ariza, 2016; Graves, 2016). The first histological evidence of sex differentiation of the gonads in chickens is shown on day 6.0, or Hamilton and Hamburger stage 29. During the primary stage of development, the gonad encases three different cell types: primordial germ cells (PGCs), steroidogenic progenitor cells, and progenitor cells (Stevant, 2018; Nefs, 2019). The remains of the daughter cells from division remains in the coelomic epithelium and mesonephros, whereas some daughter cells from division move to the genital ridge to establish functional gonadal cell lineages (Yoshino, 2016). After leaving the extraembryonic germinal crescent and moving through the circulation, primordial germ cells (PGCs) are found primarily in the medulla. After that, they multiply inside the gonads and eventually differentiate into primary spermatocytes or oocytes (Ginsburg, 1987). The mesonephros embryonic in chickens produces progenitors of supporting cells, which result in the formation of pre-granulosa and theca cells in females and Sertoli and Leydig cells in males (Estermann, 2020).

At E5.5 or HH28, there is the earliest macroscopically noticeable alteration in the bilateral gonad morphology (Guioli, 2014). Male's bipotential gonads (ZZ) develop into symmetrical testes, which are characterised by the outer cortical layers flattening and the sex cords gradually proliferating in medullae. These features provide suitable niches for PGC differentiation (Swift, 1916; Ginsburg, 1987). Then after, the germ cells inside the cords enter mitotic arrest. However, in females (ZW) is very dissimilar. According to Smith *et al.,* (2008) and Bernardo *et al.,* (2015), the inner medulla is completely unstructured and contains fluid-filled vacuoles known as lacunae that eventually experience meiotic arrest (Ukeshima, 1996). The female left gonad has a well-developed cortical layer that is filled with PGCs. Conversely, the right gonad of the female develops but does not produce a thickened cortex, and the germ cells do not undergo meiosis. These inferences are consistent with a decrease in the expression of the local Raldh2 enzyme, which synthesises retinoic acid, an inducer of meiosis for the germ cells.

The Wolffian and Mullerian ducts, two paired embryonic structures that offer ascent to the reproductive ducts of birds, are influenced by hormones (Gasc, 1981; Stumpf, 1981). Initially, both ducts are present in both sexes. Gonadal anti-Müllerian hormone (AMH), a glycoprotein hormone secreted by developing Sertoli cells, causes the paired Müllerian ducts in male (ZZ) chicken embryos to recede starting around day 9 of incubation. The male reproductive structures, the vas deferens and epididymis, are the result of the maturation of the Wolffian ducts by gonadal androgens. In females (ZW), the right Mullerian duct also recedes synchronously with the atrophy of the right gonad (Romanoff, 1960; Stahl, 1985). The gonads of females also synthesise AMH, although less so in males. The left female Mullerian duct develops into a functional oviduct, serving the left ovary. During embryonic stage, local oestrogens guard the left female duct from AMH (Josso, 1977; Hutson *et al.,* 1982). Hormones can have a long-lasting effect during early development that results in sexual differentiation. This effect is referred to as "organisational" or "activational" effect (Phoenix *et al.,* 1959; Arnold, 2009).

Avian Sex Determination

In vertebrates, sex is determined by two different types of mechanisms: environmental sex determination (ESD) and genetic sex determination (GSD) (Gamble, 2012; Bachtrog, 2014). Most reptiles, including crocodiles, turtles, and lizards, have sex-determining patterns that complement ESD (Andrews. 2008; Weber, 2020). Temperature-dependent sex determination (TSD), which maintains that the ambient temperature during incubation determines the sex of the offspring, is one of the most popular ESD processes (Charnier, 1966).

In turtles, male hatchlings from Trachemys scripta elegans eggs incubated at 26 ◦C whereas female hatchlings are produced from eggs incubated at higher temperatures (32 ◦C) (Natarajan 2016). Although GSD typically affects higher creatures, such birds and mammals (Arnold *et al.,* 2013). E4.5 is where sex determination is done (Kuroiwa, 2017). Sex differentiation of the gonads must begin during embryonic life due to gene(s) on the sex chromosomes (which are actually defined at fertilisation via sex chromosome inheritance). The mix of sex chromosomes carried by the sperm and egg during fertilisation determines the sex of the progeny (Mank, 2014). In birds, females are shown to engage in heterogamous (ZW) sex (Marshall, 2001).

Based on Chromosome

In birds, the Z dose method is a global approach for determining sex (Borsani, 1991; Ayers *et al.*, 2013; Shetty *et al.*, 2002). In birds, gonadal sex differentiation is associated with the Z (dosage effect) gene DMRT1, which encodes a transcription factor that resembles a zinc finger instead of a W-linked (ovary) factor (Major, 2017). Male birds have two Z chromosomes, while females have one. DMRT1 (Doublesex and Mab-3 Related Transcription Factor 1) is only transcribed in the urogenital system and is initially detectable at E3.5. It regulates the direction of gonadal sex differentiation (Smith, 2011; Graves, 2014; Yang, 2013; Smith, 2014). An emerging method of dose adjustment is the male hypermethylated (MHM) (Teranishi, 2001). Masculinization of female embryos results from the Z dosage technique of sex determination with overexpression of DMRT1, which is characterised by the activation of genes linked to testis development, SRY box transcription factor 9 (SOX9), and anti-mullerian hormone (AMH) (Smith, 2009; Lamberth, 2014; Lee, 2021). The expression of markers linked to female development, such as Cytochrome P450 Family 19 Subfamily A Member 1 (CYP19A1) and Fork head Box L2 (FOXL2), results in the formation of ovaries in male chickens when half-DMRT1 copy is silenced (Smith, 2009; Taylor 2021).

A dominant female determinant on the W chromosome or an inhibitor of testicular differentiation (Major, 2016; Smith, 2016; Kuroiwa, 2017). The W-linked ovary determinant gene, often referred to as WPKCI and ASW, seems to have HINTW (histidine triad nucleotide-binding protein W) as its best candidate (Hori *et al.*, 2000; Neill *et al.*, 2000). But ZZ embryos that overexpress HINTW thrive to be healthy males with two testes each (Smith *et al.*, 2009a). Situated on chromosome 4 at E4.5–E6.5, FET1 (female-expressed transcript 1) is an alternative candidate for a W-linked ovarian determinant (Reed, 2002; Sinclair, 2002). Quail's copulatory behaviour and sexual differentiation are affected by changes in oestrogen levels (Balthazart *et al.*, 2009).

Based on Molecular pathway

In males, early at E3.5, DMRT1 is detected in the medulla of the gonads, while SOX9, starting at E6.5, is involved in the development of the testis in the ZZ embryo. Z chromosome-based cHEMGN (Hemogen) function for testis differentiation (Nakata, 2013). Male paired ductus mullerian are regressed by AMH (anti-mullerian hormone), which is produced and secreted by Sertoli cells (Vigier *et al.*, 1983; Picard, 1986). However, oestrogen guards the left ductus from regress caused by AMH (Josso *et al.*, 2001).

In females, the hormone estradiol is important for the ovaries' growth (Smith, 1992). For the conversion of androgen to estradiol, AROMATASE is obtained from the medullae of the female gonads at E6.5 (Smith *et al.*, 2005). A W-linked ovarian determinant located on chromosome 4 at E4.5–6.5 is entitled FET1 (female expressed transcript 1). (Reed, 2002; Sinclair, 2002). Aromatase transcription is controlled by FOXL2 (Forkhead Box L2) (Loffler *et al.*, 2003; Wang *et al.*, 2007). In the developing ovary, aromatase and FOXL2 create loop and have a high correlation between E4.7 and E12.7 (Hudson *et al.*, 2005). R-spondin 1 (RSPO1) expression begins in embryos at E4.5 and peaked by E8.5 (Biason, 2008; Liu *et al.*, 2010; Smith *et al.*, 2008). Male and female WNT4 was detected at E4.5, while female WNT4 was upregulated around E6.5–8.5 (Kuroiwa 2017; Ayers *et al.*, 2013). A metabolite of vitamin A known retinoic acid is needed for germ cells to go through meiosis and produce oogonia (Bowles *et al.*, 2006; Andreson *et al.*, 2008). In men, cytochrome CYP26B1 inhibits this process (Trukhina, 2014). The SF1 an orphan hormone receptor family affects the initial phases of gonadal and adrenal development (Santa Barbara *et al.*, 1998).

Sex	Genes	Action
Male	DMRT1	Testes development
	SOX9	
	cHEMGN	Testes differentiation
	AMH	Regress mullerian duct
Female	ESTRADIOL	Ovarian development
	AROMATASE	Androgen to Estradiol
	FOXL2	Regulates aromatase
	SF1	Gonadal formation
	HINTW	Ovary determining
	RETINOIC ACID	Oogonia development

Primer pair specific for sex chromosome

Using primer pairs specific to a sex chromosome is a quick and easy way of sexing (Griffiths *et al.*, 1998; Ito *et al.*, 2003). Agate *et al.* (2003) claimed that the CHD Chromo-helicase DNA gene, which was identified in 1995 and is unique to domestic chickens and zebra finches, is the first gene on the W chromosome and has been utilised for sex identification in a range of animals (Ito *et al.*, 2003; Cheng *et al.*, 2006; Reddy *et al.*, 2007; Wang *et al.*, 2008; Bantock *et al.*, 2008; Vellayan, 2008). The male produced a single 380 bp band (Chd-Z) as the amplification result, while the female produced two bands (380 and 500 bp) (Ellergren, 2002).

Cell Autonomous Sex Identity

According to recent research on gynandromorphic chickens, "sex determination" in birds might begin at gonadal development and be cell independent. Based on observations from genetic and embryological studies (Scholz *et al.*, 2006; Zhang *et al.*, 2010; Zhao *et al.*, 2010). Hormones showed no effect on how gene expression affected sexual differentiation. Gene expression and embryonic development exhibit sexual dimorphisms prior to gonadal differentiation into the testes or ovaries (Alvarez *et al.*, 2010; Dewing *et al.*, 2003). Gynandromorphic chickens (gyn 5 female; andro 5 male; morph 5 shape) are bilateral sex chimaeras in which one half of the body is female and the other is male. Such occurrence is known as "genetic mosaicism" (Agate *et al.*, 2003; Zhao *et al.*, 2010). Larger wattles, combs, spurs, and breast muscles on the male side and smaller wattles, no spur, and smaller breast muscles on the female side are characteristics of gynandromorphs. This occurrence is caused by sex hormones, which are anticipated to flow to both sides of the body. In fact, ZW cells predominated on the female side, while ZZ cells predominated on the male side, it was revealed. According to some theories, sex determination in birds is cell autonomous, which means that each "cell knows its sex" cos of the complement of sex chromosomes. According to the inheritance of sex chromosome theory, sexual differentiation and sex determination are determined by genetic elements that are cell autonomous.

Mechanism of Avian Sex Reversal

Sex reversal is attributed to birds' acute sensitivity to variations in sex hormone levels (Balthazart, 2009). The mechanisms of sex determination and differentiation in birds are intimately associated with the evolutionary process; diapsid reptiles, which evolved 150 million years ago, are the ancestors of crocodiles, lizards, and birds (Smith, 2004). In eutherian mammals, gonadal sex differentiation can arise even without steroidogenesis and seems to be unaffected by sex steroid hormones (Hu, Mc 2002). Bird sex differentiation occurs in an extra-maternal domain and has characteristics in common with lower vertebrate sex differentiation. Therefore, it is plausible they are incapable of withstanding fluctuations in exogenous oestrogen concentrations, which is not usual in normal hatching conditions. Thus, extra-maternal embryogenesis's biological characteristics and the evolutionary

Types of Avian Sex Reversal

There are four types of avian sex reversal which includes

a) Natural/ Spontaneous: due to pathological condition by DDT, DDE, DEHP, MEHP, Nitrobenzene
b) Experimental/ Induced: due to sonic vibrations (male-to-female) and hormonal therapy (male-to-female by estrogen/ aromatase), (female-to-male by aromatase inhibitors/ ER modulators)
c) Environmental: due to environmental temperature in Australian bush turkey
d) Transplant treatment: by endogenous hormone

Spontaneous/Natural Sex Reversal

In chicken flocks, the socioeconomic structure of the population can affect an individual's sexual orientation (Godwin, 2009; Lamm, 2015). For instance, in a flock of chickens without a rooster, a hen may undergo sex reversal in order to preserve population reproduction (Major, 2016). Diseases are a primary source of sex reversal, and this is an adaptive modification that emerges during the long-term evolutionary process. Hermaphroditism (presence of functional ovarian and testicular tissues) or pseudo hermaphroditism (coexistence of both male and female sexual accessory organs) is a pathological condition that causes sex reversal in birds. This condition includes ovarian atrophy or regression, ovarian cysts or tumours, and adrenal diseases (Drescher, 2007; Jacob, 2000).

The development of an ovarian tumour causing arrhenoblastoma in female birds (Hughes, 2008) alters the birds' phenotypic and sex hormones (Bigland and Graesser, 1955). Ovarian follicular atrophies spurred on by Arrhenoblastoma result in a decrease in egg output. There have also been reports of ovarian cysts, tumours, and adrenal hypertrophy causing sex reversal in people and animals. In these cases, the left ovary regresses while the remaining right ovarian tissues multiply as ovotestis (Jacob and Mather, 2000). According to Dillard *et al.* (2008), Leydig cells release enough testosterone to block the effects of female sex hormones. However, as aromatase is mostly mis-expressed in extragonadal tissues, this disease-mediated sex reversal may not have an impact on gonadal shape. Pesticides such as 1, 1-dichloro-2, dichlorodiphenyltrichloroethane (DDT), and dichlorodiphenyltrichloroethane (DDT), 1, 1-dichloro-2, 2-bis (4-chlorophenyl) ethylene (DDE), Di-(2-ethylhexyl) phthalate (DEHP), mono-2-ethylhexyl phthalate (MEHP) and nitrobenzene have carcinogenic effect which may facilitate tumours in ovary (Xu *et al.*, 2010).

Experimental/Induced Sex Reversal

In avian species, granulosa cells that compose the follicular cavity and the inner envelope of ovarian follicles synthesise oestrogen. Both placenta and corpus luteum also produce estrogens. Leidig cells in the testicles and the adrenal cortex synthesis a small magnitude of such hormones (Dzhafarov *et al.*, 2010). Estrogens enter cell nuclei through the ERα and Erβ receptors, which are located in the kidney, liver, adipose tissue, and gonads. Before sexual differentiation, both sexes' gonadal cortex expresses oestrogen receptor alpha (ERα) (Trukhina, 2014).

According to Owens and Short (1995), the pathological destruction or removal of a female bird's gonad due to disease may cause an abrupt change in sex in an adult bird. It can be hindered by treatment including such aromatase inhibition (Smith, 2016), where it enabled the treated female birds to exhibit spermatogenesis in adulthood (Smith, 1992; Wolff, 1959). Birds by lacking the W chromosome are unable to be female (Kuroiwa, 2017). Hormones produced in the gonads, pituitary gland, and hypothalamus are factors that determine sexual differentiation and determination. Hormones, such as progesterone, estrogens, and androgens, are the major components of cholesterol synthesis in animal species. The ratio of the first two groups of steroid hormones is crucial for normal sexual development. An aberrant development of primary and secondary sexual characteristics may result from a disease. (Dzhafarov *et al.*, 2010; Perevoschikov, 2011; Verin, 2012).

Male-to-Female Sex Reversal

Sex-reversed birds are induced by adjusting endogenous hormone levels with the use of estrogens or aromatase inhibitors (Scheib, 1983; Elbrecht, 1992). While quail eggs are exposed to oestrogen in the first half of their embryonic life (before the onset of sex differentiation) can feminize genetic males, marked by the vacuolized inner medulla and hyperproliferation of the left gonadal cortex (Scheib, 1983) and demasculinize male individuals by injecting a 17aEthinylestradiol (EE2) emulsion into E3 quail eggs. These individuals will lose typical masculine sexual behaviour and develop asymmetric testes with fewer regions of androgen-dependent cloacal glands after maturity (Halldin,

1999). The orphan nuclear receptor steroidogenic factor-1 gene (Sf1) was up-regulated during E5-7d; the double sex and Mab-3 related transcription factor 1 gene (Dmrt1) was down-regulated during E3-7d; the anti-Müllerian hormone gene (Amh) was expressed at a similar level in genetic females and sex-reversal females prior to E7d; and no expression products of the three female-specific genes Wpkci, Fet1, and Foxl2 were found in male-to-female embryos.

Secondary sexual traits also exhibit estrogen-regulated sex reversal, not only in the gonads. The feminization of feathering patterns can be achieved by injecting estradiol into the leg muscles of adult male chickens or by giving DES 0.1 mg per egg at E0, which results in a complete sex reversal from male to female (Zhou *et al.*, 2008). This can lead to changes in saddle feather length, plumulaceous segment length, and feather colour (Widelitz, 2019). However, these effects are temporary and eventually reverse with a decrease in oestrogen levels in the body. Estrogens have a major impact on the development of secondary sexual traits in adulthood as well as the differentiation of gonadal structures during embryonic stages. The outcome demonstrates that feminising male chickens to varying degrees can be achieved by treating chicken eggs (4–7 days of development) with this emulsion (Ellis, 2012; Shioda, 2021). The left gonads of these individuals progressively form female like cortical regions and fluid-filled medullae from low to high degrees of sex reversal or into ovariotestis while the characterized testicular tissues are almost lost (Odajima, 2021). However, "the effect of estrogen-mediated male-to-female sex reversal is transient". After hatching, some reversed individuals return to their typical male morphologies, while others can maintain their female phenotypes for upto a year (Smith, 2004).

Female-to-Male Sex Reversal

Female-to-male sex reversal can be driven about by injecting aromatase inhibitors (an enzyme involved in the synthesis of oestrogen) such as methotrexate and tamoxifen (a modulator of oestrogen receptors), which lower the amount of gonadal estrogens produced in avian eggs (Elbrecht,1992; Ellem, 2010). Fadrozole, an aromatase inhibitor, when applied to E3 chicken eggs can masculinize bilateral female embryonic gonads, which fail to form stratified cortexes, but develop functional medullae enclosing germ cells at E9.5 (Hirst, 2017). Aromatase inhibitors-treated chickens exhibit varying degrees of sex reversal. The gonadal cortex is reduced in highly sex-reversed individuals, and germ cells are relocated into developed medullary structures. Through tamoxifen or letrozole injections 100uL per egg, concentration 1mg/ml done into air pocket of egg at 4th day or twice on 4th and 11th day for incubation of

19days at 37.8°C and humidity 28%. Genetic sex of each embryo was defined by polymerase chain reaction (PCR) with DNA isolation (Griffiths *et al.,* 1998). Genes involved in the formation of female embryos with reversible sex, DMRT1, SOX9, and AMH expression is significantly upregulated in gonadal medullae, whereas FOXL2 and CPY19A1 are downregulated in juxtacortical medullae and gonadal cortexes, with fewer residues. In Sertoli cells, the main AMH receptor, AMH receptor type-II (AMHR2), is upregulated and co-localizes with DMRT1 (Jianbo, 2023). After hatching, the gonadal and internal structural morphology of sex-reversed chickens continues to alter. The gonads of day-old sex-reversed chickens (D1) display both tubular structures and follicles. These tubular structures differentiate into abnormal seminiferous tubules at D11 and form atypical tubules with areas of loose connective tissue at D21. In D42 hens, the left and right gonads develop into small ovotestes, containing greatly enlarged atypical seminiferous tubules and fewer normal appearing seminiferous tubules (Xiuan, 2023).

Fradozole with IGF: Synergistic Effect of Fadrozole and Insulin-Like Growth Factor-I shows completely reversed the female phenotype. Might be useful in offsetting the disadvantage of sex-reversed chicks having reduced weight gain (Toghyani *et al.,* 2013).

Avian Sex Reversal by Transplant Treatment

Gonadal grafting can be used to alter endogenous hormone secretion, resulting in sex-reversed birds. Likewise, mixed-sex chimaeras are produced when E2 female (male) sections of the presumptive mesoderm-which give rise to gonads-are grafted to replace the corresponding male (female) tissue at the same growth stage (Zhao, 2010). Therefore, artificial transplantation of exogenous tissues can affect avian sex differentiation, leading to sex reversal.

Female to Male Sex Reversal

Early extraembryonic testis grafting can completely reverse the female chick embryo's sex differentiation toward the male sex. Transplantation of E13 (HH39) chicken whole testes into E3 female chicken extra-embryonic coelom of the host, near umbilical vessels can induce gonadal sex reversal (Maraud *et al.,* 1982a). Under the stimulation of exogenous testes, the left gonad differentiates into a testis instead of an ovary, and germ cells migrate into sex cords but not experience a meiotic process. This sex reversal is irreversible. They possess two testes associated with normally differentiated male excretory ducts and their Mullerian ducts have regressed. The development of male sex characteristics such as external features, behaviour and complete spermatogenesis is proof that these cocks possess exocrine and endocrine functions akin to those of typical cocks. These cocks were "sterile," despite the fact that they could mate with female birds.

The transplant result demonstrates that, with the exception of feather colour, the phenotypic features of the strain's cock were acquired by sexually reversing the phenotype of the fowl during embryonic life: large red comb and wattles, spurs, call and disposition of the neck, saddle and tail plumage. Since they mated with normal females, their sexual behaviour similar to males but resulting eggs were unfertile. The genital tract exhibited a cock-like morphology, with two testes whose size was reduced compared with normal. Normally, a ductus deferens and an epididymis joined these testes on either side. There was no sign of Mullerian remnants.

Avian Sex Reversal by Environmental temperature

Aside from megapodes, the Australian brushturkey, there is currently no evidence that incubation temperature influences sex ratios in birds (Ann Goeth *et al.,* 2005). Temperature does affect sex ratios in megapodes, which are unique among birds because they use environmental heat sources for incubation. Australian brush-turkey at Low temperature hatches males but at High temperature hatches females. At 34 °C incubation sex ratio is 1:1 but at 32 °C more male, while at 36 °C more female.

Adjustment of Primary sex ratio

Prior to fertilisation, female birds have the option to donate either a W or Z sex chromosome to their offspring, which might significantly skew sex ratios (Krackow, 1995; Alonson-Alvarez, 2006). At both the primary and secondary levels, the adjustment occurs (before and after fertilization, respectively). The avian ovary consists of thousands of follicles that are maintained in the diploid state and contain both a W and Z sex chromosome. A selection of follicles from the initial pool are recruited 7–10 days before ovulation into an ovulatory hierarchy that is intended for ovulation. Following this, they undergo fast yolk deposition and grow exponentially in size before ovulation. In the prophase of meiosis I, every follicle is stopped until precisely. At this time, meiosis resumes and one set of chromosomes is retained in the oocyte and the other is extruded to a polar body shows incapable of developing further. At this point, the offspring's genetic sex is established (Johnson, 2000).

Mechanism of Bias

a. The W or Z chromosome is preprogrammed to be retained by oocytes before they are recruited into the pre-ovulatory hierarchy. In order to modify the sex of their offspring, females may first preferentially recruit follicles into the pre-ovulatory hierarchy. This mechanism allows female eclectus parrots (*Eclectus roratus*) may create long strings of the same sex without laying gaps (Heinsohn *et al.,* 1997).

b. Every follicle develops at the same rate, and the order of ovulation strictly follows the order of recruitment (Badyaev *et al.,* 2005). Follicle growth rates during rapid yolk deposition are determined by the sex chromosome the oocyte is programmed to retain, revealed that follicles that eventually retained a Z chromosome grew five times faster results males (Badyaev, 2004).

Progesterone levels in the blood were significantly higher in female-producing hens, precisely when sex chromosome would be segregating & reduced the number of males produced (Johnson, 2000). Only in first-laid eggs, testosterone-treated females produce significantly more male progeny by acting either early in follicular maturation during fast yolk deposition (RYD), or it could have been absorbed by the yolk and directly influenced meiotic segregation and it can influence the segregation of sex chromosomes occur through a testosterone-mediated stimulation of vitellogenesis but estradiol is likely not a potent modulator of offsprings sex ratios in birds (Goerlich *et al.,* 2009). Although the percentage of male offspring generated after mating and the levels of testosterone in Japanese quail were negatively correlated (Correa *et al.,* 2011). Numerous species undergo female-biases due to CORT, and low follicular growth rates are linked to the production of female offspring, glucocorticoid-induced inhibition of vitellogenesis. It is possible that there is a species-specific skew in the sex ratio. Directing the blood supply (Angiogenesis) toward large or tiny clusters of oocytes to regulate the size of a single follicle. A larger cluster of follicles would produce more male progeny if growth rates were faster. Additionally, there is hormonal "cross-talk" between the granulosa layer and the egg around the time of ovulation (Yoshimura *et al.,* 1994).

Avian Sex Control

Poultry industry utilizes avian sex research to solve practical production problems. Currently, billions of male hatchlings are culled at day-old globally every year, and their carcasses are either buried in soil or further processed into feed by machines. Although these techniques reduce the cost of feed but severely breach animal welfare regulations, and untreated animal carcasses have a high probability of posing a biosafety risk to human health. The development of avian sex control technology is a viable way to address the mentioned issues and increase breeding efficiency. It was inspired by gender control systems used in dairy farms. Research on the determination, differentiation, and reversal of avian sex has provided a wealth of information regarding the advancement of early sex detection and sex control technology.

The prevalence of plumage dimorphism in hummingbirds, paradise ducks, pheasants, grouse, and manakins is significant (Sibley, 1957) between 32-42% in south-east Asia and suggests that tropical areas not unique in incidence of dichromatism (Enid Rayner *et al.,* 2015). In birds, sexual dimorphism can be exhibited in size, structure, and shape, but it is most commonly observed in plumage and coloration. Typically, the male is bigger than the female, but reverse size dimorphism among the raptors, jacanas, buttonquail, and berry pickers (Swaddle, Karubian *et al.,* 2000; Kruger, 2005). Extensive plumage displays in female migratory birds are restricted, presumably due to the associated energy costs and hazards of predation (Bailey, 1978; Simpson, 2012). During the breeding season, plumage dimorphism under genetic control (ZZ in males, ZW in females) is displayed (September to January).

Avian Sex Reversal and Cell Autonomous Sex Identity (CASI)

Birds can be made to undergo sex reversal, but after they reach sexual maturity, neither the male nor the female can successfully produce viable sperm or form well-functioning ovaries (Andrew, 2016). The CASI of avian somatic cells regulate this incomplete sex reversal, which is a cellular innate sex identification that can assist individuals in maintaining their genetic sex without the influence of hormones. CASI is influenced by epigenetic variables such histone lysine methylation and DNA methylation, as well as genetic information, particularly that inherited by sex chromosomes (Xiuan, 2023).

Sexually dimorphic gene expression has been found in various tissues between male and female birds at early developmental stages when primary gonads have not been induced to differentiation, indicates the CASI is involved in organogenesis that confirms in mixed-sex chicken chimeras & gynandromorphic birds, which exhibit a significant bilateral asymmetry. In testes, donor female cells are not recruited into functional Sertoli cells instead, they are restricted to the interstitial tissue between the sex cords. Similarly, granulosa cells in ovaries cannot be formed by donor male cells. Because differentiation of these cells is verified by their genetic destiny by showing no association between GFP+ donor female cells and AMH+ host male cells in the testes or between GFP+ donor male cells and CYP19A1+ host female cells in the ovaries.

Gonadal fate is likely maintained by epigenetic factors. In embryonic female-to-male sex-reversed chickens, DMRT1's chromatin accessibility cannot be raised to a normal male level, which is consistent with its transcriptional activity. Additionally, the failure of estrogen-mediated sex-reversed chicken gonads to form in the same manner as control females' CYP19A1 DNA methylation pattern indicates that epigenetic factors play a role in the establishment of avian gonadal CASI. Through having an impact on the development of secondary sexual traits in birds the avian CASI might play a crucial role in identifying distinct sex phenotypes (Xiuan, 2023).

Role of Hormones & Genetic effects

According to the genetic sex, the embryonic gonads synthesise and produce gonadal sex steroid hormones (Tanabe *et al.*, 1979, 1983; Clinton, 200010). The development of sexually dimorphic traits is influenced by hormones. Male chickens have larger spurs, wattles, and combs than females, while females have lesser traits. Testosterone is thought to be responsible for male comb and wattle masculinization (Zeller, 1971; Shanbhag, 1996; Yoshioka *et al.*, 2010; Lambeth *et al.*, 2016a). Different species or strains appear to have different mechanisms controlling the development of leg spurs (Lambeth *et al.*, 2016a). Oestrogens, which are synthesised by the female gonad, cause female feathering, whereas testosterone is necessary for male plumage (Lindsay *et al.*, 2011). Early in follicular development, estradiol concentrations rise, but in the most mature follicles, progesterone concentrations are higher and aid in ovulation stimulation (Johnson, 2000). The follicular cells that surround the developing oocyte produce both hormones, which are lipid-soluble and readily able to reach the germinal disc (GD), which houses the genetic information (Kristen Navara, 2013).

Research Progress & Application of technology

In early years, research conducted on the relationship between the gender of the embryo and the outer shape of the eggshell and the sex of hatchlings. This research insights into the design of avian sex control systems. By using morphometric, , allantoic fluid on 7th day with 98% accuracy (hormone "Seleggt", DNA analysis "PlantEgg") and different optical (Raman spectroscopy/Molecular fingerprints - subfield of vibrational spectroscopy based on "Raman effect", Fourier transform infrared spectroscopy, time-resolved laser-induced fluorescence spectroscopy) and imaging methods, chemical signals as biomarkers (fluorescent 93% accuracy) for sex detections, magnetic resonance imaging technology at E12-13 to differentiate sex specific growth for early sex detection (Galli, 2017), embryonic heart rate at E15-20 shows (♀ > ♂), genetically engineered technology represented by CRISPR/Cas9 system. Based on the advancements in avian sex development and spectroscopic research, farms and intensive breeding industries will be able to differentiate between male and sterile eggs. This will ultimately benefit the poultry sector.

Raman spectroscopy

Raman spectroscopy uses the spectral signature of germinal or blood cells to identify the sex of an embryo in ovulation. For instance, male and female eggs can be distinguished from one another using sex-specific molecules that are extracted from the developing chicken vascular system at stages E3 or E5, when the embryos are able to withstand the effects of external stimuli and are earlier than the connection between afferent nerves and spinal cord.

Egg morphometry

Higher egg length into male in young birds & into female in old birds respectively. Higher S.I into female in old birds. Probability of Female chick increased with increased Progesterone concentration, increase in length, width, length ratio, width ratio, S.I ratio & decrease in weight, volume of eggs. Older birds with higher shape index develop into female embryo. Younger birds with higher length develop into male embryo (Kayadan, 2023), older birds with higher shape index develop into Female embryo with accuracy of 80% (Anjana, 2023) Based on ESI with 80% accuracy.

Male group: 0.297*Length + (0.018*Width) & 0.346*Length ratio + (-0.269*Width ratio) Female group: 0.162*Length + 0.122*Width & 0.137*Length ratio + (-0.003*Width ratio)

Hypereye by Egg Farmers of Ontario

It uses hyperspectral imaging to identify infertility and gender of day-of-lay eggs accuracy 97%

Genetic Switch by ONCE

Using narrowband light-emitting diodes, a genetic switch selectively activates or deactivates the light-absorbing centres in genes that determine sex. Thus, oviparous embryos' sex can be affected during the early phases of differentiation. Only offspring of the desired sex should be able to be produced on demand (females in laying hen production and males in broiler production).

Soos Technology

Invented a technique to modify the reproductive system's gene expression in genetic male embryos, transforming males into functional females with the ability to lay eggs. An AI-guided incubation system that manipulates temperature, humidity, CO2, and vibrations to change genetically male chickens into functional females by controlling the process of sex development in poultry embryos.

Odour profile

In Japanese quail by use of SPME/GCMS in Female(E8) & Male(E1). In WLH at E1-9 with Nonanal, Octanal, 6 10-dimethyl-5 6-methyl-5-hepten-2-one, 9-undecadien-2-one, decanal, 2-nonen-1-ol: (♀>♂), 2-ethyl hexanol, hexane: (♂>♀) these change with age advances but ketone group of 2-undecanone hormone linked constituent.

CRISPR/Cas9

Direct way to govern the gender of embryonic chicken by marking sex chromosomes for in ovo sex control. Produced from genetically modified hens by labelling the Z chromosome with fluorescent biomarkers, male-determined eggs can be distinguished from female-determined eggs by their fluorescence signals either prior to or during the early stages of incubation, when they mate with non-genetically modified roosters. An Israeli biotech company created the CRISPR-Cas9 technique known as eggXYt. Green fluorescent protein is used to mark the hen's Z chromosome to identify male eggs, which are distinguished by their bright yellow colour and can be detected using an electro-optical scanner but female eggs can't impact.

Research Progress	Application
Egg morphometry 80% accuracy	In Young birds(30-32wks) with 47-52gms FEMALE: Width ratio (<8.21), Shape index (<144.44)
	In Old birds(50-52wks) with 52-57gms FEMALE: Width ratio (>7.76), Length ratio (>10.38)
TeraEgg by Vital farms	Uses infrared light & complex algorithms to analyse sex, reproduction from early stage
Poultry by Huminn	Gene edit technology regulates activation of Z chromosome by Optogenetic system, uses a blue light that shines through the eggshell at the incubator "Golda chicken" in 2021The genetic change affects only the female parental Z chromosome Male embryo will cease developing in early stage of embryonic & not hatch, eliminating the need for sexing, sorting and culling

Maternal Hormones

Higher Estrogen(non-significant), Progesterone(significant) concentration shows more female embryos. Age didn't have any impact on hormone levels.

Genetic Modification

Genetic modification makes gender determination possible before incubation by genetically marking sex chromosomes (Doron *et al.*, 2017). One pure line of hybrid chicken will be modified to incorporate enhanced Green Fluorescent Protein (eGFP) from Crystal Jellyfish (Aequorea Victoria). The Roslin institute has successfully introduced eGFP, which binds to sex chromosomes. Sex specific germinal disc fluorescence patterns can be used for gender determination of young ones (Bruijnis *et al.*, 2015).

GA-BPNN Based Gender Recognition Algorithm

The genetic algorithm (GA)- backpropagation neural networks (BPNN): a non-destructive method of gender identification of chick embryos at Day4 for integrity of blood vessels in the field of machine vision with an accuracy of 89.74%. **Male embryo:** thick main blood vessels with numerous lateral vessels and few thin branches in uniform distribution. **Female embryo:** thinner main blood vessels with fewer lateral vessels and more thin branches in irregular distribution.

Mass Spectrometry by *In Ovo*, CORDIS

Ella a fully automated machine that determines the sex of an egg ensuring only females are hatched on D9 of the incubation period with an accuracy of 95%. Having unique biomarkers, high speed sampling, mass spectrometry. Like glucose, choline, valine shows (♀>♂)

CHEGGY Based on Plumage Colour

Uses Hyperspectral imaging to identify gender of eggs at E13. Based on sex linked plumage colour. ♂- silver/white, ♀- gold/brown with accuracy 95%

Critical issues & Challenges

The hatchability of eggs, the development of chicken embryos, the production of eggs, and the survival rate of laying hens shouldn't be affected by the applied technology. Since a successful gender control approach needs to increase output effectiveness. Moreover, when researching gender control measures, biosafety, food security, and animal welfare must be taken into account. These techniques need to be appropriate from a humanitarian and ethical standpoint, as well as fit within the political climate. The highly automated and easily operated technology can be applied to intense breeding.

Limitations

Male to female sex reversal is not currently achievable. Chicks whose sex is reversed from female to male do not gain enough weight. The primary mechanism by which avian CASI resists external stimuli is currently unknown. People will be afraid to consume such hormone treated chicken. National and International strict rules and regulations.

Future Perspectives

The intrinsic regulatory mechanisms amongst the genes relevant to avian sex need to be investigated. The original CASI of avian cells is the main force to resist external stimuli during the entire developmental stage, a biological characteristic that evolved over a long period of time. However, the molecular mechanism of avian CASI still remains unclear, thus warranting further studies. Future studies on sexuality should focus more on the impact of 3D chromatin (with new technology of Hi-C) interactions on gene expression and look for epigenetic modifications that truly regulate sex-related gene expression. At the meiotic segregation stage, sex ratios are adjusted through direct hormonal mechanisms or indirectly through regulation of follicular development or yolk contents. To fully understand how adjustment of sex ratios occurs in birds, we now need to take our understanding of how meiotic segregation and the extrusion of polar bodies are regulated by hormones and/or downstream mediators down to the intracellular level. Making *in-ovo* sexing technology commercially accessible through importation or partnerships with the companies

Conclusion

Sex-reversed birds are valuable for investigating avian sex determination and differentiation due to their unique sex development mechanism. Goals related to sex control include assisting in the resolution of issues like the lack of certainty surrounding elements that determine sex and obstacles to the creation of perfect systems. To locate a "piece of evidence" as soon as feasible that offers trustworthy details on the sex of embryos and work with machines to distinguish fertilised eggs that belong to a single sex. Investigate on IGF1 in female chick's body weight by inhibiting the estrogen synthesis. Investigate the formation mechanism of sex linked Volatile Organic Compounds VOCs. Avian sex reversal is uneconomical through induced technology so, dependence on sex identification and conversion into "table eggs". Dual purpose chickens are pursued by crossing by fattening & laying lines as a compromise solution with a dual focus on meat and egg production. Male chicks "STUNNY" a high protein food pet animals' technology should be investigated. Studies on intracellular level to pinpoint how hormones or mediators control the process of meiotic segregation and extrusion of polar bodies in sex adjustment. Regardless of the type of treatment used, the chicken cannot achieve complete sex reversal, even during embryonic periods due to the CASI of avian somatic cells. The alteration of hormone levels can only cause partial or temporary sex reversal in birds. Birds can't be female without the W chromosome. The goal of sex control differs from species to species. Before making any effort for development of sex control technology, it is essential to consider the biological characteristics of the species. For the successful sex reversal, timing dosage, and method of hormone treatment should be standardized. While applying the sex reversal technology for the commercial scale culture, effective population size should be taken into consideration.

Index